OFFICE OF POPULATION CENSUSES AND SURVEYS
SOCIAL SURVEY DIVISION

Adult dental health

Volume 1

England and Wales
1968 – 1978

A survey conducted by the Social Survey Division of
OPCS in collaboration with the Department of
Dental Health, University of Birmingham Dental
School for the United Kingdom health departments

J E Todd
A M Walker

London: Her Majesty's Stationery Office

ISBN 0 11 701022 7

Acknowledgments

We would like to thank everybody who helped to make this survey possible. First of all the other staff at Social Survey Division who contributed to the different stages of the survey, including all the interviewers who carried out not only their usual task of interviewing but also that of dental recording.

Our special thanks go to the dental organisers for the part they played and particularly for the smooth running of the dental training courses — a considerable undertaking involving 64 dentists and an equal number of interviewers from all over the United Kingdom. On behalf of ourselves and the dental organisers we would also like to thank all the dental examiners who took part in the survey especially for the way they adapted to the unfamiliar circumstances of conducting the survey examination in people's homes.

The practice sessions of the training courses were held at a research establishment in Newcastle and we would like to say thank you to all the volunteers from there, many of whom were examined a large number of times and also to Procter and Gamble for allowing us to use their staff time and facilities.

Finally, of course, we must thank all the informants who participated in the survey, for without their co-operation all our efforts would have been to no avail.

The dental organisers

Dr RJ Anderson
Mrs JH Nunn
Mr PS Hull
Professor PMC James
from the Department of Dental Health, University of Birmingham Dental School.

Contents

Notes on the tables

Base numbers have been given in italics. Where a base number is less than 30, statistics have not been given and this is indicated by an asterisk. A dash in a table represents a proportion of less than 0.5% or a mean of less than 0.05 or a zero value.

The varying positions of percentage signs and bases in the tables denote the presentation of different types of information. Where the percentage sign is at the head of a column and the base is at its foot the whole distribution is presented and the figures add to 100%. A percentage sign and base at the side of an individual figure signifies that this proportion of people had the attribute being discussed and that the complementary proportion (not shown in the table) did not.

1 Introduction

1.1 Background to the Survey

The first national survey of adult dental health to be carried out in this country took place in 1968[1]. This study provided basic information about the dental health of adults in England and Wales and the variation in their dental condition with particular reference to differences found between the regions. As well as providing a current picture of the dental health of adults, the 1968 survey enabled a base line to be established from which future change could be measured.

When it was decided to launch another study of Adult Dental Health in 1978, two main purposes were identified. First to ascertain whether there were any changes in adult dental health over ten years and second to provide a picture of adult dental health in 1978, which would allow the introduction of any new bench marks that had become important in the period between the surveys and that might prove relevant for future measurements of change.

Although the 1968 survey had been commissioned to provide statistics for England and Wales, in 1972 a Scottish Study[2] had also been carried out on behalf of the Scottish Home and Health Department, and by 1978 statistics for many subjects were increasingly being required on a United Kingdom basis. It was therefore decided to extend the survey to cover the UK rather than perpetuate a situation in which studies in the different countries were in a different sequence.

The sample for the survey was designed so that a certain amount of analysis could be carried out for Wales, Scotland and England separately. This entailed some over-sampling in Wales and Scotland. Since the survey was to represent the United Kingdom, part of the sample was, of course, selected in Northern Ireland, but from the outset it was agreed that no separate results would be given for Northern Ireland because to do so would require extensive oversampling*.

As with the previous dental surveys, part of the fieldwork involved a dental examination. Responsibility for the design of the methods used in the dental examination and the training of the survey dental examiners was undertaken by the Department of Dental Health of the University of Birmingham Dental School. Throughout the initial planning and launching of the survey their staff worked in close collaboration with the Social Survey Division. Proposals for the dental examination were laid

before and agreed by a dental steering committee, which comprised representatives from the commissioning departments, the community dental service and the field of dental epidemiology.

1.2 Outline of the methodology

A sample of approximately 7250 individuals was selected from the Electoral Register and supplemented using a sampling technique carried out at the fieldwork stage to include 16 and 17 year olds and other adults who were not on the Register. The sample covered the whole of the UK with proportionately more people selected from Scotland and Wales than from England and Northern Ireland. The fieldwork involved an interview and a dental examination, the latter being conducted by a team of dentists seconded from the community dental service. The dental team attended a one week training course before the fieldwork where they were introduced to the format of the survey examination and learnt to work to the survey dental criteria. Calibration and recalibration exercises were carried out before and after the fieldwork to give a measurement of examiner variability.

All the selected individuals were asked to take part in an interview in their homes and those with some natural teeth were asked at the end of the interview to take part in a dental examination a few days later. The exclusion of the edentulous from the dental examination was the one major departure from the overall scheme adopted in the previous surveys in which all people had been asked to take part in the examination. The survey dental examination was carried out in the informant's home by one of the seconded dentists, accompanied by an interviewer acting as the dental recorder.

The interview contained questions about the informants' dental experiences including their visits to the dentist and the types of treatment they had received. People with natural teeth were asked about their attitudes towards dental care and total tooth loss while those who had dentures were asked about their experience of wearing dentures and their attitudes towards having them. Some topics were covered in exactly the same way as in the previous studies while others were approached slightly differently and a few completely new topics were introduced.

Many features of the dental examination were necessarily very similar to the examination used in the 1968 study. This was particularly so for information recorded about the condition of natural teeth. Rather different examination approaches were used with respect to the condition

---

* In fact a dental survey based on the same criteria and techniques as have been used in this study was carried out in Northern Ireland at the end of 1979.

of the gums, the relative positions of the teeth present and for information about dentures.

A small pilot study was conducted in January 1978 and the main fieldwork took place in April, May and June 1978.

1.3 The Sample
A detailed description of the sample and the method used to select it will be found in Appendix A. However, a general description of the main features of the sample will clarify why some of the analysis procedures used throughout the report are necessary.

The survey required a sample of adults aged 16 and over living in private households. People living in institutions were excluded because of the difficulties involved in sampling and interviewing them. This group had been excluded from the other dental enquiries for the same reasons. The sample was to be spread throughout the whole of the United Kingdom.

The most important factor determining the size of the sample was that it needed to be large enough in England and Wales to detect any major changes that had occurred over the previous ten years and that the sample selected in Scotland needed to be large enough to conduct analyses similar to those carried out in the 1972 Scottish survey and to make some sound comparisons between the two surveys over six years.

Another consideration affecting the size of the sample was that in the 1968 survey, Wales had been grouped with the South West of England for regional analysis, since the sample size was not large enough for both regions to stand alone. With hindsight this grouping was not seen to be particularly appropriate since, from a dental viewpoint, the two areas are very different. Although for comparisons over the last ten years this original grouping has to be retained, it was agreed that, when looking at dental conditions in 1978, Welsh figures would be presented separately, which meant obtaining a sample large enough to permit such analyses.

There were, of course, constraints on how large the sample could be; one of the determinants being the number of dental examiners used and another, inevitably, the cost. Two changes from the basic scheme used in the 1968 survey were introduced to maximise the use of our resources. The first change was the exclusion of the edentulous from the survey dental examination, which allowed an increased sample size to be selected without the need for increasing the number of dental examiners. The second was the selection of proportionately more people in Wales and Scotland than in England, which facilitiated separate analyses without increasing the size of the sample required in England. In the 1968 survey we had used a two stage sampling process, selecting parliamentary constituencies at the first stage and individuals at the second. Constituencies were chosen as the first stage units because they were 'not so small as to be unduly influenced by the activities of one dental practice within them but were

small enough to avoid using too much of the examining dentist's time in travelling between selected people'[3]. This was just as true in 1978 and so the same basic design was adopted.

Consideration of all the above mentioned factors led to the selection of 39 constituencies and about 4700 individuals from England, 20 constituencies and about 1750 individuals from Scotland and 12 constituencies and about 650 individuals from Wales. In Northern Ireland 160 individuals were selected but using a slightly different scheme (see Appendix A). In Scotland, proportionately 3.3 times as many people were selected as in England while in Wales the equivalent figure was 2.4. Consequently if figures for the four countries are simply added together Scotland and Wales would be over represented. Thus all the figures for Scotland and Wales have to be downweighted by factors of 1/3.3 and 1/2.4 respectively when presenting United Kingdom results.

The downweighting procedure necessary for arriving at the correct UK figures has consequences for the base figures of tables. One is that the rounding of decimal places in the downweighted base figures leads to rounding errors and thereby slight inconsistencies in base numbers. The other effect occurs where figures are presented separately for Scotland and Wales and also for the UK. In these cases we have chosen to present the unweighted (actual sample size) figures for Scotland and Wales while the UK figure will, of course, include the downweighted values for Scottish and Welsh figures.

1.4 The survey dental examiners
The survey information was collected using two methods: an interview and a dental examination. The Social Survey Division maintains a field force of interviewers but, of course, has no readily available team of dental examiners. The previous dental surveys had used dental examiners from a variety of sources, and for the 1978 study the community dental service was asked to provide the necessary examiners.

The sample was designed so that in England each constituency would provide the workload for one dental examiner. In Wales and Scotland however, the constituencies needed to be grouped in order to do this. Most of the constituencies selected in Wales were paired on a geographical basis, so that dental examiners could cover a pair of constituencies. Since the Scottish sample contained a higher number of people per constituency than the Welsh one, it was thought that the workload resulting from two constituencies might be too great for one dental examiner to carry out in six weeks. Therefore, individual constituencies which covered a large area, and would involve more travelling, were allocated one per dental examiner and smaller ones were paired and allocated to dental examiners who were asked to be available for nine weeks rather than six. In the event however, most examinations had been completed by the end of the six week field period.

By using the community dental service we ensured that all

the dentists were working fairly near to home which was a method of minimising the overall costs. In order to achieve this, we had to ascertain in which Area Health Authority or Health Board each selected constituency was situated. We then contacted the relevant authorities and asked if they would release a dentist from his normal duties to carry out the survey work in their area. As constituency and health area boundaries are not aligned, there were a few cases where the selected constituency fell in two different health areas.

In these cases we asked the area containing the larger part of the sample to second a dentist and informed the other area that the survey would be taking place. There were also some instances where more than one constituency was selected from one health authority so that more than one dentist was needed from that area. In most cases these areas seconded the number of dentists needed. All but two areas were able to release a dentist to work on the survey and for the two who were not, neighbouring health authorities seconded dentists to carry out the survey work. This resulted in a team of 62 dental examiners and a list of the survey dental team will be found in Appendix B.

Ideally all the survey dental examiners working on the survey should have attended the same training course so that variation in the data collected could not possibly be attributed to any variation in the method of training. However, with a large sample of people to be examined in a relatively short time, the number of dental examiners needed to complete the fieldwork meant that it was impossible to train them all on one course.

The dental examiners were allocated to one of two consecutive training and calibration courses according to the area in which they would be working, to ensure a regional mix at each training course. All the other work to do with the content and management of the two training courses was carried out by the Department of Dental Health of the University of Birmingham Dental School and a detailed description of this will be found in Appendix B.

1.5 The survey interviewers
The interviewers working on the survey were drawn from Social Survey Division's team of interviewers who are trained by the division and who work on the range of surveys which comprise the continuous programme of survey research carried out by the division. The interviewers were specially briefed for the dental questionnaire and trained to be dental recorders about a week before the dental examiners were ready to start the fieldwork. This gave the interviewers an opportunity to carry out their first interviews and so be able to arrange some dental examinations for the survey dental examiner to conduct as soon as he had completed the training course.

Each dental examiner worked with between two and four interviewers. Although we arranged for the dentist to meet one of his interviewers during the dental training course, we could not arrange for him to meet them all and so we asked the dentist and all his interviewers to meet on

the first working day, have a practice session together and make their arrangements for the fieldwork. As the dentist was to be working with a number of interviewers, we organised a basic rota system nominating particular days that were to be worked with each interviewer. This basic rota was amended by each team as required, but was a very necessary starting point since interviewers needed to know while they were interviewing at what time they could make appointments with the public to return with the dentist for the dental examination.

Part of the interviewer's role at the examination visit consisted of 'shielding' the examiner from too close an involvement with the informants since most of the dental examiners had never conducted home examinations before. The examination was conducted in a coded form so no information was passed to the informant and the interviewers were instructed to try to prevent or divert dental queries being directed at the dental examiner. On the whole this worked well particularly as the informant already knew the interviewer from the preceding interview.

The method of carrying out the dental examination and the equipment used is described in Appendix B.

1.6 The Response
In all sample surveys the number of people who agree to participate is very important, but in this one it was particularly so since there were two stages where non-response could be introduced. In the initial introduction to the survey the interviewers stressed the importance of all people taking part, since it is always a problem in dental surveys that people who have lost all their natural teeth may not see the relevance of the survey to themselves, and so may decline to take part. When asking the informants if they would take part in the dental examination, every effort was made to ensure the smallest possible loss at this stage and the interviewers were given a list of points to mention in order to encourage people to participate. Overall we achieved interviews with 89% of the individuals selected and dental examinations with 86% of those eligible (Table 1.1).

Table 1.1   The response achieved

a) Sample of addresses		
Number of addresses selected	7266	
Withdrawn (obvious institutions)	113	
	7153	
No person for interview at address	878	
Effective sample of addresses	6275	
b) Co-operation achieved at the interview		
		%
Interview obtained	5967	89
Refusal	529	8
Non-contact	183	3
Total people selected from 6,275 addresses	6679	100
c) Co-operation achieved at the examination		
		%
Dental examination obtained	3495	86
Refusal at end of interview	398	10
Refusal at second call	96	2
Non-contact at second call	93	2
People interviewed who had some natural teeth	4082	100

3

The sampling method used for this survey provided a representative sample of individuals but was initially based on addresses (see Appendix A for a detailed description of the sampling technique). Individuals were selected from 6,275 of the original sample of 7,266 addresses selected for the survey. Those addresses which did not yield anybody for interview comprised mainly institutions, empty or demolished properties and those where the selected individual had moved away while the rest of the household remained.

With the addition of a sample of the 16 and 17 year olds and other people who were not registered but were found to be living at the selected addresses, a total of 6,679 people were eligible for interview. Of these, 89% were interviewed, 8% declined to take part and 3% could not be contacted by the interviewer either because they were always out or because they were away for the period of the fieldwork.

Only people who had some natural teeth were asked to take part in the dental examination. Among the people who were interviewed, 4,082 had some natural teeth. A dental examination was obtained from 86% of these people while 10% said at the end of the interview that they did not wish to take part and a further 2% declined to participate when the interviewer re-called with the dental examiner. There were only 2% of people who initially agreed to take part but were not contacted when the interviewer returned. The size of this group was kept small by ensuring that the interval between the interview and the examination appointment was a short as possible and also by giving the informant an appointment card so he knew when to expect the interviewer and examiner.

1.7 Contents of the report
The results of the 1978 Adult Dental Health Survey are presented in two volumes. The first volume includes the analysis of the dental condition of adults in England and Wales in 1978 compared with the situation in 1968. The second volume portrays the current dental health situation for adults in 1978 for the whole of the United Kingdom and includes results shown separately for Scotland and Wales. The second volume also includes material about topics which were introduced for the first time in 1978 or were collected differently in 1978.

References
[1] Gray, Todd, Slack and Bulman *Adult Dental Health in England and Wales in 1968* HMSO 1970
[2] Todd and Whitworth *Adult Dental Health in Scotland 1972* HMSO 1974
[3] Gray *et al* op.cit. page 4

2 The interview and dental examination

2.1 Introduction

In determining the content and design of both the questionnaire and the dental examination, we had to strike a balance between, on the one hand, the need to produce results comparable to those from the 1968 survey and, on the other, the need for changes suggested by the hindsight of ten years and the experience of two other national dental surveys. A major change in the design of the dental examination was, of course, necessitated by the decision to examine only dentate adults in 1978, whereas all adults, including those with no natural teeth, had been eligible for examination in 1968. No such major changes were implemented for the interview stage of the survey.

2.2 The Questionnaires

There are two main sub-divisions in the analysis of survey dental data: people who have some natural teeth and those who have lost them all. However, from the point of view of collecting the data, informants are best divided into three broad categories: those who have only natural teeth, those who have lost all their teeth, and those who have a combination of their own teeth and dentures.

To interview all these people using the same questionnaire would be very cumbersome since there are obviously different topics which are appropriate to each group. So, as with the previous surveys, we used three different interview questionnaires with a brief introductory questionnaire which established which of the three main documents the interviewer should use.

The questionnaire for people with only natural teeth was designed to establish the informants' dental attitudes and their dental experiences. More specifically we wished to ascertain their attitudes towards dental treatment, the appearance of their teeth, wearing dentures and becoming edentulous. Questions relating to their dental experiences covered the types of treatment received both as a child and as an adult, their most recent visit to the dentist and, visiting the dentist in general, and, finally, a section on the NHS system of dental charges to assess their knowledge, experience and opinions of the current system.

The questions covering dental experiences were also included in the questionnaire for people who had lost all their natural teeth. However, the major part of their interview concerned total tooth loss and denture wearing. These informants were asked in some detail about the loss of the last of their natural teeth both from the factual point of view and what they had felt about it. We asked briefly about their denture wearing experience prior to becoming edentulous and in more detail about their present denture wearing. This latter section included questions on when the dentures were worn, whether they caused any difficulties and what the informant thought about their appearance.

The questionnaire for people who wore dentures in conjunction with natural teeth consisted of all the appropriate questions from the other two questionnaires plus a few which were relevant only to those with some natural teeth who also had dentures.

In all of the questionnaires many of the questions were identical to those used in 1968, in particular the one which established dental attendance pattern since this is an important variable in the analysis. Some were designed to obtain similar information but using a more compact form and some topics were tackled in a completely different way.

The interviews for people with only natural teeth and for people who were edentulous took about half an hour while the interview for people who had partial dentures took about forty-five minutes.

2.3 The Dental Examination

The detailed dental criteria used in the survey dental examination are presented in Appendix B, but it is useful at this point to give a general description followed by a discussion of the differences between this examination and the one used in 1968.

The 1978 survey dental examination consisted of four main parts: the condition of the teeth, the condition of the soft tissues, the orthodontic condition and, for people who had them, some details about dentures. In assessing the condition of the teeth, each tooth space was identified and the presence or absence of the tooth recorded. Teeth which were present but unrestorably decayed were recorded as such and crowned teeth were also identified at this stage. The potential tooth space left by each missing tooth was examined and classified according to the current situation as being filled by a denture, filled by a bridge, remaining as a space or having disappeared through other teeth closing together. Information was then recorded about the condition of each surface of every standing tooth (including those which were unrestorably decayed or crowned). A surface could be coded as sound, decayed, filled (with an amalgam, gold, or synthetic filling) or decayed and filled. At the computing stage these codes were summarised to give the overall condition of each tooth.

The information concerning the soft tissues around standing teeth was recorded for the six segments of the mouth. The presence or absence of soft debris, calculus, gingivitis (in a mild or severe form) and periodonitis was noted.

In the next part of the examination, an assessment was made of whether the teeth were crowded (again looking at the six segments of the mouth), the size of the overjet and overbite (the first measured in millimetres, the second in terms of the fraction of the lower teeth covered by the upper teeth), and finally whether the upper front teeth rested in front of the lower lip when the mouth was closed. For people who had no dentures, the dental examination ended at this point although the examiner still had to record the existence of any dental anomalies but this was usually completed after the examiner and interviewer had left the informant.

The part of the examination concerning denture wearing comprised an assessment of whether the denture was adversly affecting the mouth and a description of the denture itself. It must be remembered that only dentate people were eligible for examination so the criteria for the section on adverse effects concerned only those effects related to natural teeth and the support of natural teeth. The denture description, which was recorded separately for upper and lower jaw dentures, covered whether the denture was full or partial, of what it was made, its type (toothborne, tissueborne or both), whether it was broken or dirty, whether in the examiner's opinion it needed replacement and the number of gum margins it surrounded.

2.4 The examination technique

As in the case of the criteria, a more detailed description of the examination technique will be found in Appendix B. The survey examination was carried out in the informant's home by a dental examiner seconded from the community service, who had been specially trained for the survey, with an interviewer acting as a dental recorder. The survey examiners were advised not to discuss the condition of the informant's teeth with the informant and the examination was recorded in a coded form to prevent any breach of dental etiquette.

Much emphasis was placed on designing an examination technique which would impose on informants as little as possible. The informants were asked to sit in a high backed chair, if one was available, and the examiners were supplied with hand-held examination lights. The equipment was limited to simple probes, a mirror, a small rule to measure overjet and sterilizing solution. The sterilizing solution was carried in a container which could also hold probes and mirrors. The examiners were asked to supply a sponge or cloth and towel so that they could clean their hands without imposing on the informant.

The survey dental examination itself took about 5 minutes but the length of the whole call, including introductions, setting up the equipment, settling the person to be examined and drawing the visit to a close, took something nearer 15 minutes.

2.5 Comparison of this dental examination with the 1968 survey dental examination

Two major features distinguish the 1968 and 1978 survey dental examinations. One is the decision to exclude the edentulous from the 1978 dental examination (with the consequence that all the 1978 examination details about dentures refer only to dentures worn in conjunction with natural teeth). The other is that a different approach was used to collect information concerning the soft tissues in 1978. (See detailed examination criteria given in each report.) This change was introduced because with hindsight and greater experience the soft tissue data from the 1968 survey were not thought to be entirely satisfactory so this was one item where comparability was forsaken in order to achieve better results.

Other differences between the two examinations were either in the form of modifications which could be translated back to the 1968 examination for comparisons or additions to the amount of information collected. One modification was the different approach to bridges and crowns. In 1968 these had been coded and presented in the analysis as a separate group. In 1978 bridges were included as one category of teeth which were missing while crowns were included with the teeth which were present and so had their surfaces separately coded. Thus in 1978 it was possible to record the fact that a crown was decayed. Thus in the presentation of the UK data in Volume II, the number of decayed teeth includes decayed crowns and the number of missing teeth includes spaces which have been bridged. However, these are minor changes and the original grouping has been used in the comparison of the 1968 and 1978 data in Volume I.

Two additions were made in 1978 to the amount of information collected in the survey dental examination. One concerned the orthodontic condition and the other the state of the tooth space where teeth were missing. The first was introduced because it was felt important to build up continuity between basic orthodontic data as collected on children's studies and the dental state of adults: while the second was a direct result of the experience of analysing the 1968 survey. The 1968 report states that 'in future... we would record for each missing tooth the size of the gap. Secondly, we would record for each missing tooth whether the space had ever been filled with a denture...(these items of information) are very necessary if any attempt is to be made to estimate the need and provision of dentures for partial tooth loss'.[1] In fact, we recorded the size of the gap only if a denture or bridge was not occupying the tooth space at the time of the examination.

The changes in design that have taken place have enabled us to retain features for which we wanted to measure change, to modify those measures which could be improved and to introduce appropriate new topics. As was mentioned earlier, a detailed description of the criteria, examination technique and dental examiner training methods will be found in Appendix B.

Copies of all the documents used are reproduced at the end of this report.

Reference

[1] Gray *et al. Adult Dental Health in England and Wales in 1968.* HMSO 1970

3 Measuring change in dental health

One of the main purposes of the 1978 Adult Dental Health Survey was to provide data for comparison with the results of the earlier dental surveys carried out in 1968 in England and Wales and 1972 in Scotland. We have already mentioned that the requirement to measure change was one of the major factors taken into account in determining sample size and that as many as possible of the 1968 dental criteria were retained so as to make comparisons over time feasible.

There are, however, some other factors that affect comparisons made over time and before we go on to present the results we discuss their effects on the interpretation of the data.

Firstly it must be remembered that the surveys were based on random samples of individuals and the samples were drawn independently from one another, that is they are two separate snapshots of the situation. The design did not incorporate any element of seeking information from the same people after a certain amount of time had elapsed. Thus the two sets of survey results are subject to two independent amounts of sampling error and this will need to be taken into special consideration when the data are presented for sub-groups where the sample size is small. When account is taken of the effect of sampling error in those cases it may happen that apparent changes over time are judged not to represent real differences.

Sample surveys are not only subject to sampling errors but they are also subject to possible biases introduced because not everyone selected for the sample was prepared to co-operate. It is usually very difficult to estimate with any kind of precision what the effect of non-response has been and many studies have to fall back on the assumption that the non-responders were not so very different from the responders. However, when two sets of results relating to the same topic are available at different times the later information may lead to a reappraisal of the initial interpretation.

Another factor that has to be borne in mind is that the surveys represent snapshots of the population at the time that they were carried out, but birth, death and migration will have changed the population structure over the period concerned. If some of the attributes being studied, for example whether or not people have any natural teeth, are closely associated with the age structure of the population, then an apparent change in dental health of the population might be accounted for solely by the change in age distribution. This could be so not only for

the country as a whole but also within the different regions.

Table 3.1 shows the age distribution for England and Wales in 1968 and 1978 and the equivalent survey figures. The table shows that 19% of the population were aged 65 and over in 1978 compared with 17% in 1968. So the population structure has changed slightly. The survey figures show that in 1968 the survey was deficient in the youngest age group and that the 1978 survey was less deficient in this respect. Although these differences are not large enough to have any serious effect at the national level, they have to be kept in mind when analysis is conducted for sub-groups of the data such as regional analyses. From the point of view of population changes and sample deficiencies the most accurate comparisons to make are those within age groups.

Table 3.1 Age distribution in the population and in the dental health surveys in 1968 and 1978 (England and Wales)

Age	Population figures		Survey figures	
	1968	1978	1968	1978
	%	%	%	%
16-24	18	17	13	16
25-34	16	19	18	18
35-44	16	15	19	17
45-54	17	15	16	16
55-64	16	15	17	15
65-74	11	12	12	12
75 or more	6	7	5	6
Total	100	100	100	100

As can be surmised from the preceding paragraphs a certain amount of caution is needed when making an assessment of whether or not real change has taken place, as clearly there are sources of variation which may bear no relation to dental health at all.

Another area of concern when measuring change over time using only two observations is that it is very easy to imply that all of the change which has occurred over a ten year period has been the result of actions taken in that ten year period. This is clearly not the case. For example, if there is a reduction in the number of people aged 35-44 who have no natural teeth, the reasons for this may be connected with changes in dental attitudes and practices today, but may also be connected with the level of conservative dentistry available to young people twenty years earlier. It must therefore be borne in mind that the cause of change does not necessarily occur in the same time period as the manifestation of that change.

4 Total tooth loss in England and Wales

4.1 Total tooth loss: 1968 and 1978

A simple but nevertheless useful dental indicator for the community is the proportion of people of all ages who have no remaining natural teeth, that is, in dental terms, the proportion of people who are edentulous. A substantial part of the 1968 report considered this proportion and its variation among sub-groups within the population; for example, people in different age groups, people in different regions, people in different social classes and so on.

As the state of being edentulous is irreversible, total tooth loss is a very valuable dental indicator when looking at change over time because there is a limit on the amount of change which can take place. Some people lose all of their natural teeth when they are quite young and have many years of their life still ahead of them. They will therefore number among the edentulous for perhaps fifty years. This means that the proportion edentulous in the community cannot be drastically reduced overnight since all the people already edentulous will continue to be so for the rest of their lives. For example, in the 1968 survey there were some people in the age group 16 to 24 who had already lost all their teeth, so even if from 1968 onwards not one more person was rendered edentulous it would still take till about the year 2028 before the total population was dentate. We therefore cannot expect to find very large improvements for the whole population in the ten year period between 1968 and 1978. Although, of course, for particular age groups considerable changes can have occurred.

People who had no natural teeth and were in their forties in 1968 will, in 1978, still be among the edentulous but will be in their fifties. During that ten year period, however, more people in the group will have become edentulous and so, one way of analysing the data, is by investigating cohorts of people and measuring the level of change that has taken place, over the last ten years. Another way of looking at the changeover time is to compare the level of total tooth loss among a particular age group, say people in their forties now, with the levels for people in their forties ten years ago. Some of the most interesting results will, of course, be for those age groups where the actual incidence of total tooth loss is greatest (Table 4.1).

The 1978 survey found that 29% of adults of all ages were edentulous. This figure compares favourably with the 37% found to be edentulous in 1968. For each age group the situation was better in 1978 than in 1968. This was only marginally the case for people aged 65 and over but in these age groups the levels of edentulousness were largely affected by previous dental history. The greatest change between 1968 and 1978 occurred among the middle age

Table 4.1 Total tooth loss for different age groups in 1968 and 1978

Age	Proportion of people with no natural teeth			
	1968		1978	
16-24	1%	395	—	635
25-34	7%	515	3%	755
35-44	22%	550	12%	690
45-54	41%	475	29%	637
55-64	64%	494	48%	625
65-74	79%	343	74%	493
75 and over	88%	160	87%	235
All ages	37%	2932	29%	4075*

*   *Includes 5 people for whom age was not known.*

groups. For example, among 35-44 year olds in 1968, 22% had lost all their teeth compared with 12% in 1978. If we look at the 1978 results for the same cohort, that is those aged 45-54, we see that 29% of them were edentulous which is a markedly improved situation from people of a similar age in 1968 among whom 41% had lost all their teeth.

Being edentulous is a dental state that cannot be reversed. It is therefore possible to use the 1968 data to predict what the level of edentulousness would be in 1978 if people were becoming edentulous at the same rate as they had been in the past. It is also possible to predict from the 1968 data what the level of edentulousness would be in 1978 if, over the intervening ten years, there had been a complete cessation of people having full clearances. Such estimates provide outer limits against which the actual position reached, as measured by the 1978 survey, can be assessed*.

For example, Table 4.1 shows that 41% of 45 to 54 year olds in 1968 had no natural teeth, so if there had been no reduction in the level of edentulousness over time then the expected level of total tooth loss among people aged 45 to 54 in 1978 would also be 41%. If, however, no-one had become edentulous in the ten years between the surveys the expected level of edentulousness for the 45 to 54 year olds in 1978 would be 22%, that is the level for the 35 to 44 year olds in 1968.

Thus the results presented in this chapter not only provide a direct comparison between the 1968 and 1978 surveys, but also present the 1978 data within the estimated limits of there having been no reduction over the ten years in the level of edentulousness and the maximum reduction that could have occurred.

The diagram (Figure 4.1) shows that the levels of total tooth loss among the younger age groups were closer to

---

* It is of course possible for the situation to be one of deterioration over time but in practical terms it would seem sufficient to present the results in terms of no change or some positive change.

Figure 4.1 Total tooth loss for different age groups

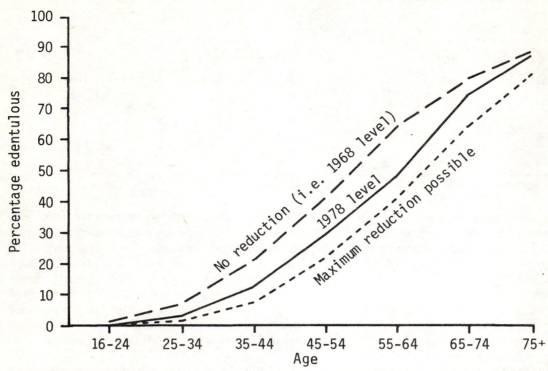

the estimated maximum reduction than those among the older age groups. This was presumably due to older people being closer to becoming edentulous through having either a higher number of missing teeth or a greater likelihood of tooth loss through periodontal disease, so that any change, in dental attitudes or treatment would have less effect on the rate at which full clearances were taking place among this group than among people in the younger age groups.

Just as the levels of total tooth loss for each ten year age group can be combined to give an overall level for the 1968 and 1978 survey results so can the values for the estimated maximum reduction. Thus we find that, given the situation in 1968, the lowest possible overall level of edentulousness that could have been achieved in 1978 was 23%. Since this value was dependent on nobody at all having been rendered edentulous since the 1968 survey, the actual figure of 29% for 1978 represents a sizeable improvement in the dental condition of adults in England and Wales over the last ten years.

4.2 Regional variation in total tooth loss

One of the most striking findings of the 1968 dental health survey was the large regional variations found with respect to every aspect of dental health. Table 4.2 shows whether the improvement seen overall for England and Wales was apparent in every region.

The 1978 survey found in each region a level of total tooth loss which was less than that found by the 1968 survey. However in the Midlands and East Anglia the difference was not large enough to be statistically significant (31% compared with 34%). For the three other regions the size of the difference seemed to be related to the 1968 level of edentulousness with the largest decrease being found in the region which had the highest level of total tooth loss: the North. In 1968 45% of people in the North had lost all their teeth compared with 33% in 1978. Even among the people with the lowest level of total tooth loss, those in London and the South East, the proportion edentulous dropped from 28% to 21%.

Table 4.2 Total tooth loss by region for people in different age groups in 1968 and 1978

Age	Proportion of people with no natural teeth																			
	The North				Wales & the South West				Midlands & East Anglia				London & the South East				England and Wales			
	1968		1978		1968		1978		1968		1978		1968		1978		1968		1978	
16-24	2%	125	—	171	—	49	1%	103	1%	95	—	146	—	126	—	215	1%	395	—	635
25-34	15%	136	6%	218	7%	72	3%	127	4%	114	4%	168	2%	193	1%	242	7%	515	3%	755
35-44	32%	159	16%	187	26%	77	13%	117	20%	123	10%	161	13%	191	9%	225	22%	550	12%	690
45-54	55%	139	32%	167	33%	60	31%	118	48%	103	34%	152	27%	173	21%	200	41%	475	29%	637
55-64	73%	150	62%	173	74%	80	55%	116	55%	105	47%	153	55%	159	31%	183	64%	494	48%	625
65-74	81%	109	87%	128	89%	61	75%	98	82%	62	78%	122	69%	111	60%	145	79%	343	74%	493
75 and over	93%	46	93%	60	88%	32	75%	49	89%	27	93%	61	84%	55	83%	65	88%	160	87%	235
No reduction			45%	864			43%	431			34%	629			28%	1008			37%	2932
1978			33%	1105			32%	729			31%	965			21%	1276			29%	4075*
Max. reduction †			30%				26%				24%				16%				23%	

Includes 5 people for whom age was not known.

†*These figures were calculated by applying the 1968 proportion edentulous to the 1978 base for each age cohort.*

Table 4.3 Total tooth loss for different age groups and sexes in 1968 and 1978

Age	Proportion of people with no natural teeth					
	Male		Female		Both sexes	
	1968	1978	1968	1978	1968	1978
16-24	1% 183	— 316	1% 212	— 319	1% 395	— 635
25-34	6% 253	3% 330	8% 262	4% 425	7% 515	3% 755
35-44	16% 282	9% 346	28% 268	14% 344	22% 550	12% 690
45-54	36% 208	24% 314	44% 267	33% 323	41% 475	29% 637
55-64	61% 252	41% 312	66% 242	56% 313	64% 494	48% 625
65-74	78% 147	72% 219	80% 196	76% 274	79% 343	74% 493
75 & over	88% 57	86% 74	88% 103	87% 161	88% 160	87% 235
No reduction		33% 1382		40% 1550		37% 2932
1978		24% 1912		32% 2163		29% 4075*
Max. reduction†		20%		27%		23%

Includes 5 people for whom age was not known.
† *See footnote to Table 4.2*

Table 4.2 also shows the estimated maximum reduction in total tooth loss possible for each region. In all the regions except for the Midlands and East Anglia the proportion of edentulous people in 1978 was more than half way towards this maximum.

To see if there was any explanation for the comparative lack of change in the Midlands and East Anglia we compared the age distributions for the two surveys and found that in 1978 there was a greater proportion of elderly people in this region than there had been in 1968. This change reflected an actual change in the population structure. Although the calculation of the estimated maximum reduction in total tooth loss took into account varying age distributions we saw in Figure 4.1 that the elderly were further from achieving the maximum than were the younger adults, and this will have contributed in part to the 1978 level of 31% edentulous.

The largest differences within age groups for each region were among the 55 to 64 year olds for London and the South East and Wales and the South West (55% down to 31% and 74% down to 55% respectively) but in the North and Midlands and East Anglia the largest difference was found among the 45 to 54 year olds. With regard to the absence of any large overall improvement in the level of edentulousness among people in the Midlands and East Anglia the proportion of edentulous 55 to 64 year olds in 1968 is of particular interest. The relationship of this figure (55%) with the proportion edentulous in the other age groups in 1968 and 1978 appears to be very different from the equivalent relationships in the other regions. It is different in such a way to suggest that the sample selection of this age group in the Midlands and East Anglia could perhaps have produced an artificially low estimate of the proportion edentulous which would, in turn, have led to a low overall estimate of total tooth loss for the Midlands and East Anglia in 1968.

The result of all the regional changes over the last ten years was to reduce slightly the overall difference between all four regions and to reduce considerably the differences between the North, Wales and the South West and the Midlands and East Anglia. About one in three adults living in each of these areas was found to be edentulous compared with one in five people living in London and the South East.

4.3 Variation in total tooth loss between the sexes

The report of the first dental health survey stated that women in the North accounted for a large part of the regional difference in total tooth loss[1] although there were also quite substantial regional differences among the men. We now go on to investigate how the levels of edentulousness have changed over the last ten years for men and for women with particular reference to the effect this has had on the overall levels in the regions.

In 1968 we found 33% of men were edentulous compared with 40% of women. This difference was still apparent in 1978 although the level of total tooth loss had decreased for both sexes (to 24% for men and 32% for women). The variation with respect to age was similar to that seen ten years ago with women having lost their teeth earlier in their lives than men but with the levels of edentulousness equalising among men and women aged 65 or more. For women the largest decrease in the proportion of people who had lost all their teeth was among the 35 to 44 year olds while for men the largest reduction was among the 55 to 64 year olds. This variation has transferred the largest difference between men and women in the levels of edentulousness from among the 35 to 44 year olds to the 55 to 64 year olds.

The estimated maximum reduction in total tooth loss, given the 1968 data, was 20% for men and 27% for women so that the survey results of 24% for men and 32% for women show a similar rate of improvement for the two sexes over the last ten years. This is demonstrated in Figure 4.2 which shows the two survey values and the theoretical lowest possible value for each age group. Once again it is evident among both sexes that the younger groups were closer to achieving the maximum reduction in total loss than were the older age groups.

Both men and women have shown a similar amount of improvement in their levels of total tooth loss over the last ten years, while there has been variable improvement in the different regions so we go on to examine the relative changes among men and women within the different regions (Table 4.4).

In Wales and the South West and the Midlands and East Anglia the degree of improvement among the men was very similar to that among the women. In the North,

Figure 4.2 Total tooth loss for different age groups and sexes

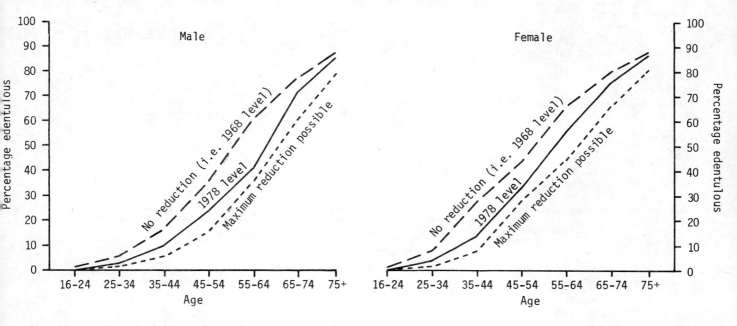

Table 4.4 Total tooth loss for different age groups, sexes and regions in 1968 and 1978

Age	Proportion of people with no natural teeth							
	The North				Wales & the South West			
	Male		Female		Male		Female	
	1968	1978	1968	1978	1968	1978	1968	1978
16-24	2% 57	— 90	3% 68	— 81	* 25	2% 49	* 24	— 54
25-34	12% 74	7% 113	19% 62	4% 105	9% 32	1% 52	5% 40	4% 75
35-44	25% 81	16% 82	40% 78	15% 105	11% 37	14% 56	40% 61	13% 61
45-54	47% 53	25% 91	60% 86	39% 76	* 23	33% 50	35% 37	30% 68
55-64	70% 76	53% 77	77% 74	70% 96	69% 36	47% 61	77% 44	65% 56
65 and over	84% 58	88% 78	85% 97	89% 110	92% 40	70% 50	85% 53	78% 97
No reduction	39% 399		51% 465		39% 193		46% 238	
1978	29% 531		37% 574		28% 318		35% 411	
Max. reduction†	24%		35%		21%		31%	

Age	Midlands & East Anglia				London & the South East			
	Male		Female		Male		Female	
	1968	1978	1968	1978	1968	1978	1968	1978
16-24	— 45	— 80	2% 50	— 66	— 56	— 97	— 70	— 118
25-34	— 55	2% 62	8% 59	6% 106	3% 92	1% 103	1% 101	1% 139
35-44	16% 69	5% 95	26% 54	17% 66	12% 95	4% 113	15% 96	13% 112
45-54	45% 60	30% 67	51% 43	36% 85	22% 72	15% 106	31% 101	28% 94
55-64	57% 53	40% 80	54% 52	55% 73	53% 87	27% 94	57% 72	36% 89
65 and over	78% 36	82% 82	89% 53	84% 101	71% 70	61% 83	76% 96	71% 127
No reduction	30% 318		38% 311		27% 472		30% 536	
1978	27% 467		35% 498		16% 596		24% 680	
Max. reduction†	21%		27%		14%		18%	

† *See footnote to Table 4.2*

however, the proportion of edentulous women showed a larger decrease over the last ten years than that of men (51% to 37% compared with 39% to 29%). In fact, the 1978 level of total tooth loss for women in the North nearly reached the estimated maximum reduction. This was also true for the men in London and the South East where the level in 1968 was 27% edentulous, in 1978 was 16% edentulous and the estimated maximum reduction possible was 14%. We found that the men in the South East showed a greater improvement than the women.

Thus the two largest rates of improvement were found among the two most extreme groups, those that had the highest level of tooth loss in 1968, women in the North, and those with the lowest level of total tooth loss in 1968, men in the South East. It clearly follows from this that men in the South East must in 1978 have retained their position of having the lowest level of total tooth loss in England and Wales. However, despite the large improvement among the women in the North they maintained their position of being the group with the highest level of edentulousness and Table 4.4 also shows that it was the women in this region who accounted for it having the largest overall improvement.

The result of all these changes was that the difference bet-

Table 4.5 Total tooth loss in England and Wales by household social class

Household social class		Proportion of people with no natural teeth					
		1968			1978		
Professional	I	15%	112 ⎫		11%	282 ⎫	
Intermediate	II	31%	503 ⎬ 27%		22%	805 ⎬ 21%	
Skilled non-manual	IIInm	25%	335 ⎭		26%	379 ⎭	
Skilled manual	IIIm	34%	1074	34%	28%	1382	28%
Semi-skilled non-manual	IVnm	47%	100 ⎫		36%	132 ⎫	
Semi-skilled manual	IVm	46%	419 ⎬ 46%		33%	494 ⎬ 37%	
Unskilled	V	47%	153 ⎭		47%	222 ⎭	
Housewife		68%	181		53%	190	
Others*		38%	55		28%	188	
All social classes		37%	2932		29%	4075	

* *Students, unemployed and not classifiable*

Table 4.6 Total tooth loss in England and Wales by household social class and age-groups

Age	Proportion of people with no natural teeth											
	I, II, III nm				III manual				IV, V		All people	
	1968		1978		1968		1978		1968	1978	1968	1978
16-24	1%	131	—	198	2%	167	—	220	— 76	1% 143	1% 395	— 635
25-34	2%	177	1%	302	7%	206	5%	277	13% 109	6% 134	7% 515	3% 755
35-44	12%	179	7%	272	24%	241	14%	258	34% 109	14% 127	22% 550	12% 690
45-54	31%	170	18%	250	43%	177	34%	222	49% 114	38% 128	41% 475	29% 637
55-64	51%	150	39%	226	64%	161	51%	210	72% 144	61% 142	64% 494	48% 625
65-74	65%	101	65%	160	87%	84	76%	152	80% 87	85% 110	79% 343	74% 493
75 or more	81%	42	81%	56	92%	38	84%	44	91% 33	95% 62	88% 160	87% 235
No reduction			27%	950			34%	1074		46% 672		37% 2932*
1978			21%	1466			28%	1382		37% 848		29% 4075*
Max. reduction†			16%				21%			31%		23%

* *These totals include the housewife, student, unemployed and unclassifiable categories which were not included elsewhere in the table.*
† *See footnote to Table 4.2.*

ween the proportions of edentulous men and women in each of the four regions in 1978 was almost identical to that seen for England and Wales as a whole while in 1968 there had been considerable variation between the regions.

4.4 Total tooth loss and household social class

The final factor considered in the 1968 survey was the social class of the household in which the informant lived, which was determined by the occupation of the head of the household. We had found considerable variation in the levels of total tooth loss for people in different social classes in 1968 and Table 4.5 shows this was still the case ten years later.

Once again, people in social class I had the lowest level of total tooth loss and people in the 'Housewife' group the highest. This latter result was not unexpected since households headed by housewives tend to be single person households comprising elderly widows. What was slightly unexpected however was that although the majority of groups showed a decrease in the level of total tooth loss similar to that seen overall, there was no apparent change among people in classes III non-manual and class V. However, an analysis of the age distribution within these two social class groups showed that in both cases there was a greater proportion of elderly in the 1978 sample than in the 1968 sample. This difference in age structure in the two samples did, in fact, reflect what appeared from other sources[2,3] to be an actual change in the population.

Table 4.6 shows that the level of edentulousness among the grouped social classes had decreased fairly evenly among the I, II, III non-manual and the III manual groups while people in groups IV and V showed a slightly larger decrease in their level of total tooth loss. In fact comparison with the estimated maximum reduction possible showed that people in the lowest social class group were closest to achieving this result. This large improvement originated mainly from the 35 to 44 year olds in groups IV and V, among whom 34% had lost all their teeth in 1968 compared to only 14% in 1978.

We have seen that there was slightly more improvement in the level of total tooth loss among people in social classes IV and V than among people in other classes. It was also shown earlier that the 1978 survey found a level of edentulousness in the North and in Wales and the South West which was closer to the maximum reduction than in the other two regions. Taking these two results together, it is not particularly surprising to see that people in the North in classes IV and V show the largest decrease in the proportion of edentulous people (Table 4.7). In Wales and the South West, however, the largest decrease were found among people in classes III manual (from 41% to 27%) and for this region the 1978 proportion of edentulous people in classes IV and V was less than halfway towards the level achieved by the maximum reduction. There was very little variation in the size of the change between different social classes in either London and the South East or the Midlands and East Anglia. Thus, neither the actual level of edentulousness nor the size of the improvement could be explained by social class differences within region.

Table 4.7 Total tooth loss in England and Wales by region and social class

	Proportion of people with no natural teeth			
	I II IIInm	III manual	IV V	All social classes
	The North			
No reduction	29% 241	43% 335	57% 218	45% 864
1978	24% 341	35% 384	38% 273	33% 1105
Max. reduction	19%	29%	36%	30%
	Wales & the South West			
No reduction	36% 144	41% 153	49% 90	43% 431
1978	25% 259	27% 248	44% 140	32% 729
Max. reduction	21%	22%	30%	26%
	Midlands & East Anglia			
No reduction	29% 178	28% 240	41% 162	34% 629
1978	23% 292	30% 381	37% 227	31% 965
Max. reduction	18%	20%	31%	24%
	London & the South East			
No reduction	21% 387	26% 346	37% 202	28% 1008
1978	16% 574	18% 369	31% 208	21% 1276
Max. reduction	11%	16%	24%	16%
	England & Wales			
No reduction	27% 950	34% 1074	46% 672	37% 2932
1978	21% 1466	28% 1382	37% 848	29% 4075
Max. reduction†	16%	21%	31%	23%

† *See footnote to Table 4.2*

4.5 Total tooth loss before the age of thirty

When the first national adult dental survey was conducted in 1968 a great deal of interest was expressed in whether there was any indication of an improvement in community dental health over time. As there was no previous bench mark from which progress could be measure, analysis relating to change could only be carried out within very strict constraints. Some measure of change over time was possible if a dental health indicator could be defined which could be seen to reflect dental change over time and was known for different age cohorts in the sample.

It was argued that early total tooth loss, say before the age of thirty, was a suitable indicator of change in that any improvement should lead to it declining over time and, being an age-specific event, it was a variable which could be determined for all persons over the age of thirty. It was thus possible to look at different age cohorts and see whether early total tooth loss was, in fact, on the increase, on the decrease, or stationary.

This proved to be a very useful part of the analysis in 1968 and although base line data now exist to measure change between 1968 and 1978 it is still useful to carry out an analysis of early total tooth loss for different cohorts as it gives an indication of change over a much longer period than ten years.

Table 4.8 presents the analysis of the 1978 data with respect to total tooth loss before the age of thirty. The data was derived from an interview question which asked people who had lost all their natural teeth how old they were when that happened. For those who were in the oldest age groups and had lost their teeth when they were young, we were asking them to recall over a long period of time. Thus, it is likely that the cohorts of older people will contain more unreliable data than the cohorts of younger adults. We have presented the results in five year bands for the younger cohorts, where memory will have played less of a part, but in ten year bands for the older cohorts.

Table 4.8 Total tooth loss before the age of thirty as measured in 1978

Age in 1978	Proportion of all people who had lost their teeth before thirty		
	Both sexes	Male	Female
30-34	3% 363	3% 156	3% 207
35-39	5% 373	4% 188	6% 185
40-44	7% 317	4% 158	10% 159
45-54	8% 637	6% 314	9% 323
55-64	9% 625	8% 312	10% 313
65-74	12% 493	11% 219	12% 274

The 1978 survey shows a continuous decline in the proportion of people who lose all their natural teeth before they are thirty. The values for the cohorts aged 30-34 and 35-39, which are the people who have entered the analysis since 1968 and thus represent the current rate of early tooth loss, suggest that early tooth loss is still declining.

The data from the 1978 study and that from the 1968 study provide us with two independent estimates of the level of early total tooth loss for some of the cohorts. By translating the current age of the cohorts into what they were ten years ago we can compare these two estimates (Table 4.9).

None of the differences between the surveys amounts to more than could occur by chance with two independent random samples.

4.6 Conclusions

In terms of total tooth loss the results show that there has been an improvement over the last ten years in the dental condition of adults in England and Wales. In 1968 37% were found to be edentulous compared with 19% in 1978. This general improvement was evident among most of the sub-groups of people we investigated.

The very large differences in the level of total tooth loss

Table 4.9 Total tooth loss before the age of thirty as measured in 1968 and 1978

Age in 1968	Proportion of all people who had lost their teeth before thirty					
	All		Male		Female	
	1968 Survey	1978 Survey	1968 Survey	1978 Survey	1968 Survey	1978 Survey
30-34	5% 260	7% 317	4% 129	4% 158	5% 131	10% 159
35-44	7% 550	8% 637	4% 282	6% 314	11% 268	9% 323
45-54	8% 475	9% 625	6% 208	8% 312	9% 267	10% 313
55-64	11% 494	12% 493	10% 252	11% 219	12% 242	12% 274

13

found between the regions in 1968 have also diminished, there being no difference between any of the regions except London and the South East which still had a substantially lower level of edentulousness. The proportions of edentulous men and women had both decreased over the ten year period and by approximately the same amount so that in 1978 there were still proportionately more edentulous women than men. This was also true for the social class groups among whom most had a lower level of total tooth loss than in 1968 but with the variation with respect to social class still being much in evidence.

References
[1] Gray *et al. Adult Dental Health in England and Wales in 1968*. HMSO 1970.
[2] OPCS. Census 1971. *Economic Activity part IV.* HMSO 1976.
[3] OPCS. *General Household Survey 1978.* Additional data.

5 Changes in the circumstances of total tooth loss and in partial denture wearing

5.1 The circumstances of total tooth loss
In 1968 we looked at the circumstances of total tooth loss among those people who had lost the last of their natural teeth at some time since the setting up of the National Health Service, that is during the period 1948 to 1968. About 55% of all the people who were edentulous in 1968 had lost their teeth during that period. The appropriate comparisons to make using the 1978 survey data are those relating to people who become edentulous during the period between the two surveys, that is between 1968 and 1978. About 20% of the people found to be edentulous at the time of the 1978 survey had lost their teeth during this period.

There were two particular features of the circumstances of total tooth loss that were of interest for comparison. Firstly, whether or not people who became edentulous had worn partial dentures* prior to losing the last of their natural teeth, and secondly how many teeth were in fact extracted at full clearance.

When looking at the survey results in detail it must be remembered that the comparisons being made do not exactly represent the complete picture of full clearances between 1948 and 1968, and between 1968 and 1978 for only people still surviving at the end of each period will be

selected in the sample. This is, of course, more of a problem for data relating to the longer period.

Table 5.1 shows that among people who became edentulous in the period 1968 to 1978 the overall proportion who had partial dentures prior to losing the last of their natural teeth was very similar to the comparable figure for people interviewed in 1968 about the preceding twenty years, in both cases about half the people becoming edentulous had previously had some kind of denture.

The number of teeth extracted at full clearance was shown in 1968 to be related to whether or not the person had previously worn a denture. Table 5.2 shows for the two periods being compared where extracted and whether the person already had a denture.

The 1968 survey also showed that a relatively large proportion of people who had become edentulous had lost 21 or more teeth at full clearance, but that very few dentate people had 21 or more unrestorable teeth, and the Scottish study showed that few people had large numbers of teeth in need of extraction for periodontal reasons. Thus previous survey findings suggested that there was considerable latitude in terms of both dentist and patient attitude towards the retention of natural teeth and the provision of dentures. Given that over the last ten years there has been a decline in the proportion of people becoming edentulous, then in terms of the circumstances surrounding total tooth loss, one might similarly expect some reductions in the manifestation of lack of regard for natural teeth. Table 5.2 bears this out. Among people who lost the last of their teeth in the interval between the surveys, only a quarter lost 21 or more teeth, whereas the comparable figure for the earlier period was a third. Although there was a slight reduction in the numbers of teeth extracted among people who had a denture before full clearance, most of the change occurred for people who had no previous denture experience. Among this group full clearances involving 21 or more teeth were carried out in 38% of cases for those who lost their teeth in

---

* It needs to be made clear that when we refer to people who have partial dentures, this includes anyone who has some combination of natural teeth and dentures. In dental terms, a denture is classified as partial or full for each jaw, but in survey terms a person who is described as a partial denture wearer may in fact have a full upper denture only.

Table 5.1 Whether or not people who had become edentulous in the relevant periods had previously had partial dentures

Whether had partial dentures	Became edentulous 1948-68	Became edentulous 1968-78
	%	%
Previously had partial dentures	49	51
Did not	51	49
Total	100	100
Base	*532*	*227*

Table 5.2 The number of teeth extracted on the last occasion according to whether or not the person was partially dentured at the time

Number of teeth extracted on the last occasion	Previously partially dentured		Not previously partially dentured		Both groups	
	Became edentulous 1948-68	Became edentulous 1968-78	Became edentulous 1948-68	Became edentulous 1968-78	Became edentulous 1948-68	Became edentulous 1968-78
	%	%	%	%	%	%
1-11	53	62	12	25	32	44
12-20	33	28	34	37	34	32
21 or more	14	10	54	38	34	24
Total	100	100	100	100	100	100
Base	*264*	*115*	*268*	*112*	*532*	*227*

the more recent period compared with 54% of cases between 1948 and 1968.

Thus although the proportion of people who had some kind of partial dentures before having full dentures did not appear to have changed, the proportion having full clearances involving very large numbers of teeth had declined and this was especially so among those who lost all their teeth with no previous denture experience.

Although the overall proportion of people with partial dentures remained at a similar level, there were some variations within different age groups (Table 5.5). In the younger age groups, the proportion was lower in 1978 than it had been in 1968, and, conversely, from the age of 45 onwards, a higher proportion had partial dentures in 1978 than was so in 1968.

The first accession of partial dentures was thus occurring

Table 5.3 Proportion of people in different regions who had previously had partial dentures or had 21 or more teeth extrated on the last occasion

Became edentulous	The North		Wales & the South West		Midlands & East Anglia		London & the South East		England & Wales	
	Proportion who had previously had partial dentures									
1948-68	44%	197	54%	85	50%	112	51%	138	49%	532
1968-78	41%	70	52%	46	40%	53	71%	58	51%	227
	Proportion who lost 21 or more teeth on last occasion									
1948-68	41%	197	26%	85	35%	112	29%	138	34%	532
1968-78	36%	70	25%	46	19%	53	12%	58	24%	227

When we investigated these results by region (Table 5.3), we found very little change in the North, which in 1968 had the lowest proportion of people who had partial dentures at full clearance and the highest proportion who lost 21 or more teeth. In London and the South East, however, the proportion of people who had a partial denture prior to becoming edentulous had increased between the two relevant time periods while the proportion who lost large numbers of teeth had decreased.

5.2 Partial denture wearers
In Chapter 4 we presented the survey findings relating to the proportion of people in the community who had lost all their natural teeth. A smaller proportion of people were found to be in this state in 1978 than had been the case in 1968 (Table 5.4). Chapter 4 did not investigate, however, whether the high proportion of people who were found to be dentate include relatively more or fewer people with partial dentures.

Table 5.4 Dental status in 1968 and 1978

Dental Status	1968	1978
	%	%
Natural teeth only	41	51
Partial dentures	22	20
Edentulous	37	29
Total	100	100
Base	*2932*	*4075*

The results show that overall it was not a large rise in partial denture wearing which offset the reduction in tooth loss, but rather it was that the proportion of people with only natural teeth had risen substantially.

Table 5.5 Proportion of all adults with partial dentures by age

Age	Proportion with partial dentures			
	1968		1978	
16-24	7%	395	5%	635
25-34	22%	515	15%	755
35-44	29%	550	25%	690
45-54	34%	475	35%	637
55-64	23%	494	30%	625
65-74	13%	343	17%	493
75 and over	6%	160	9%	234
All ages	22%	2932	20%	4075*

* *Includes 5 people for whom age was not known*

later and it also seemed possible that the transition from partial dentures to full dentures was being deferred. If these types of changes were occurring then one would expect them to manifest themselves in the pattern of partial dentures that people had and we go on to look at this next.

5.3 The pattern of partial dentures
The pattern of dentures worn by a partially dentured person can be a full denture for one jaw opposed by natural teeth, a full denture opposed by a partial denture or partial dentures only in one or both jaws.

We were interested to see whether the pattern had changed at all between 1968 and 1978. Table 5.6 shows the proportion of partially dentured people who had each combination of dentures in 1968 and 1978.

Table 5.6 The pattern of partial denture wearing in 1968 and 1978

Denture pattern		Adults with some natural teeth who have (had) of denture	
Upper jaw	Lower jaw	1968	1978
		%	%
Full denture	None	17 } 34	13 } 29
Full denture	Partial denture	17	16
Partial denture	Partial denture	23 } 61	23 } 65
Partial denture	None	38	42
None	Partial denture	5	4
Partial denture	Full denture	—	1
None	Full denture	—	1
Total		100	100
Base		*562*	*839*

The proportion of people with partial dentures who had a full upper denture but no lower denture had decreased from 17% to 13% while the proportion who had a partial upper denture but no lower denture had increased. Thus again there seems to be evidence of a reduction in large scale extractions and an increase in preserving what can be retained. This may be due in part to current changes in attitudes and dental values and may also be due to the investment in restorative dentistry over the past few decades which has prolonged the life of natural teeth. Clearly the results regarding the natural teeth need to be closely scrutinised in later chapters to see if the likelihood of such hypotheses can be confirmed.

In the previous section there was evidence that fewer younger people had partial dentures in 1978 so we look next to see whether the changing pattern of dentures also varied with age.

Table 5.7 shows that, as one would expect, the people in the older age groups had a heavier involvement with dentures than those in the younger age groups. In the middle age group, that is people aged 35 to 54, there was, however, a significant reduction in the proportion of partial denture wearers in 1978 who had a full upper denture, and a consequent increase in the proportion with partial upper dentures compared with 1968. Thus, once again, the data suggest that in the middle age groups there was a reduction in the amount of treatment involving large scale extractions.

Table 5.7 The pattern of partial denture wearing for different age groups

Denture pattern		Adults with some natural teeth who have (had) a denture					
Upper jaw	Lower jaw	16-34		35-54		55 and over	
		1968	1978	1968	1978	1968	1978
		%	%	%	%	%	%
Full denture	None	6 }12	9 }14	18 }37	13 }26	22 }46	14 }40
Full denture	Partial denture	6	5	19	13	24	26
Partial denture	Partial denture	21 }82	11 }80	23 }57	23 }68	26 }51	27 }52
Partial denture	None	61	69	34	45	25	25
None	Partial denture	5	6	6	4	2	4
Partial denture	Full denture	1	—	—	1	1	3
None	Full denture	—	—	—	1	—	1
Total		100	100	100	100	100	100
Base		*129*	*149*	*289*	*393*	*144*	*293*

6 People with natural teeth

6.1 Introduction

We have seen that over the last ten years both the level of total tooth loss and the proportion of large scale full clearances have decreased while the pattern of partial dentures has changed in the direction of there being fewer full upper dentures than was the case in 1968.

Each of these changes suggests that there may be a greater dental awareness in the community and that there is, in some sense, a greater value being placed on natural teeth. It is, therefore, of particular interest to investigate whether any changes have taken place in the condition of natural teeth. The changes already mentioned could affect the state of natural teeth in several ways. For instance, if there is a general improvement in the awareness of people to dental problems of all kinds, then any change seen among the edentulous and those with dentures might be expected to manifest itself in appropriate improvements for natural teeth. If, however, the changes in the condition of the groups already studied reflect merely a change with respect to dentures, rather than dental health generally, then the residual effect of people not having full clearances or full upper dentures could be to worsen the average condition of natural teeth.

6.2 The condition of natural teeth in adults

The condition of the teeth of the people who took part in the survey was established during the survey dental examination. As we have explained in Chapter 2, the criteria and design of the dental examination were formulated in such a way as to introduce the modifications suggested by ten years hindsight, while at the same time maintaining the facility to produce results comparable to the 1968 survey examination results.

Thus, as was the case in 1968, there were eight categories into which each of the thirty-two tooth positions could be classified:
i) sound and untreated
ii) crowned

iii) filled (otherwise sound)
iv) filled and decayed
v) decayed, not previously treated, but restorable } actively decayed
vi) decayed, not restorable
vii) bridged
viii) missing (not bridged)

These categories were mutually exclusive and covered the whole range of conditions in which natural teeth might be found.

Table 6.1 shows that in 1978 the average number of missing teeth among dentate adults had decreased by 1.3 since 1968. Thus, not only were more people keeping some natural teeth, but the people who had some natural teeth were retaining more of them than ten years ago. They also had, on average, one more filled tooth, and the average amount of decay was slightly lower than in 1968.

The changes seen overall were reflected among both the men and the women although there was a larger decrease in the average number of missing teeth for the women than for the men. In fact, this larger decrease resulted in there being no significant difference between men and women in the average number of missing teeth. However, since the other changes were of similar sizes, women still had more filled teeth on average than men and men still had more sound and untreated teeth.

Although the distribution of the average number of teeth in the different conditions might, at first sight, suggest that conclusions can be drawn about levels of both treatment and disease, such conclusions may be very misleading. In the 1968 report attention was drawn to the fact that the kind of dental treatment people had received could override the survey assessment of disease levels. In the survey dental examination the assessment of decay was visual, thereby recording a fairly advanced state of decay. A dentist seeing a patient in his surgery may diagnose decay at a much earlier stage and fill the teeth con-

Table 6.1 Mean number of sound, decayed and treated teeth among adults with some natural teeth

Tooth conditions	Average number of teeth in each condition					
	Male		Female		Both sexes	
	1968	1978	1968	1978	1968	1978
Sound & untreated	13.3	13.6	12.3	12.9	12.8	13.2
Crowned or bridged	0.1	0.3	0.1	0.3	0.1	0.3
Filled (otherwise sound)	6.2	7.0	7.5	8.5	6.8	7.8
Filled & decayed	0.7 ⎫	0.8 ⎫	0.6 ⎫	0.7 ⎫	0.7 ⎫	0.7 ⎫
Decayed, not previously treated but restorable	1.4 ⎬2.6	1.0 ⎬2.2	0.9 ⎬1.8	0.7 ⎬1.6	1.1 ⎬2.2	0.9 ⎬1.9
Not restorable	0.5 ⎭	0.4 ⎭	0.3 ⎭	0.2 ⎭	0.4 ⎭	0.3 ⎭
Missing*	9.8	8.9	10.3	8.7	10.1	8.8
Total	32.0	32.0	32.0	32.0	32.0	32.0
Base	*858*	*124*	*836*	*124*	*1694*	*2486*

* Throughout this report the missing includes teeth which were missing for any reason (See Criteria in Appendix B).

cerned. For such teeth the survey dental examination will record the restorative treatment provided. However, for people who do not seek regular dental advice, a similar level of decay could not be detected by the survey visual assessment and the teeth would be recorded as sound and untreated.

Conclusions about the different forms of treatment received and current gross decay are therefore more reliable than any interpretation of the estimated overall disease level. We therefore take the major treatment categories (and active decay) and examine them separately in more detail.

6.3 Missing teeth

Since every tooth lost is a step towards edentulousness, we start by looking at the variation in the average number of missing teeth. We have already seen that dentate men and women had, on average, fewer missing teeth at the time of the 1978 survey than was the case ten years earlier. We suggested at the beginning of the chapter that one of the effects of the changes seen in earlier chapters might be to make the condition of teeth among the dentate worse, but this did not seem to be the case with respect to missing teeth. Table 6.2 shows the results in more detail giving the average number of missing teeth for different age groups.

the regions that had the greatest decrease in the proportion edentulous. This might have worsened the average position with respect to missing teeth among the dentate, if some of the people who, in earlier times, might have become edentulous tended to have a fairly high number of missing teeth.

A comparison of the average number of teeth in the various conditions provides a good overall summary of the changes over the last ten years but for some purposes it is, perhaps, more useful to investigate the distribution of the actual number of teeth in each condition. It is particularly interesting to look at the extremes of such distributions, for, if change is taking place, it is often in the marginal situations that its impact can be detected.*

For example, people may have anything from no teeth missing to 31 teeth missing before they become edentulous. Any community that wishes to aim towards a major lifetime reliance on natural teeth would want the distribution of missing teeth to be shifting towards zero. Although the average gives some indication of this, a clearer understanding of how things are changing and what actions might be desirable can be obtained from more detailed information. So as not to overwhelm the reader with results we present the proportion of people

Table 6.2 Mean number of missing teeth among dentate people in different age groups in 1968 and 1978 by sex.

Age	Male		Female		Both sexes	
	1968	1978	1968	1978	1968	1978
16-24	4.9 *171*	4.7 *283*	5.4 *200*	4.7 *284*	5.2 *371*	4.7 *567*
25-34	7.3 *226*	5.9 *271*	7.6 *219*	6.2 *370*	7.5 *445*	6.0 *641*
35-44	10.0 *221*	8.2 *277*	11.0 *175*	9.4 *251*	10.5 *396*	8.8 *528*
45-54	13.7 *124*	12.0 *210*	15.2 *133*	12.7 *173*	14.5 *257*	12.3 *383*
55 and over	17.1 *116*	16.3 *203*	17.5 *109*	15.7 *164*	17.3 *225*	16.0 *367*
All ages	9.8 *858*	8.9 *1244*	10.3 *836*	8.7 *1242*	10.1 *1694*	8.8 *2486*

There were fewer missing teeth on average among dentate people of every age group. The largest difference was found among the 45 to 54 year olds who in 1968 had, on average, 14.5 teeth missing compared to the 1978 figure of 12.3 missing teeth. This figure was, of course, affected by the fact that there were fewer partial denture wearers with full upper clearances than had been the case in 1968. The larger overall change in the numbers of missing teeth among the women than among the men resulted from a much larger decrease in the average number of missing teeth for the women aged 45 or more.

In terms of change in the regions, Table 6.3 shows that there was a more substantial reduction in the average number of missing teeth in London and the South East and in the Midlands and East Anglia than in the North, while in Wales there was, in fact, no change at all. We saw earlier that the North and Wales and the South West were

Table 6.3 Mean number of missing teeth among dentate people in different regions in 1968 and 1978.

Regions	1968	1978
The North	10.3 *436*	9.0 *620*
Wales & the South West	9.5 *213*	9.5 *434*
Midlands & the East Anglia	10.4 *373*	8.7 *590*
London & the South East	9.9 *672*	8.2 *842*

with fewer than 6 missing teeth, and the proportion with 18 or more missing teeth. Obviously an improvement in dental condition is represented by an increase in the first and a reduction in the second.

Figure 6.1 shows for dentate people of different ages and from different regions the proportion of people who have a few teeth missing and the proportion who have a large number missing. The results are compared for 1968 and 1978.

There were some fluctuations in the figures because the sample size of some of the sub-groups was rather small. In terms of the proportion of people with fewer than 6 missing teeth, there had been an improvement in this proportion for all regions for nearly all age groups. This was particularly the case for London and the South East where the 1968 levels were already as high as the other

* It is often the case with national survey data that other researchers at later times wish to use the information as base line indicators for more specialised projects, we have therefore presented a considerable amount of data at the end of this chapter for reference but have limited the text presentation to a much more restricted range. Where survey results have been presented in graphical form the figures on which they are based are given in the tables at the end of this chapter.

Figure 6.1 Proportion of dentate adults in different age groups and regions with fewer than 6 missing teeth and of those with 18 or more missing teeth

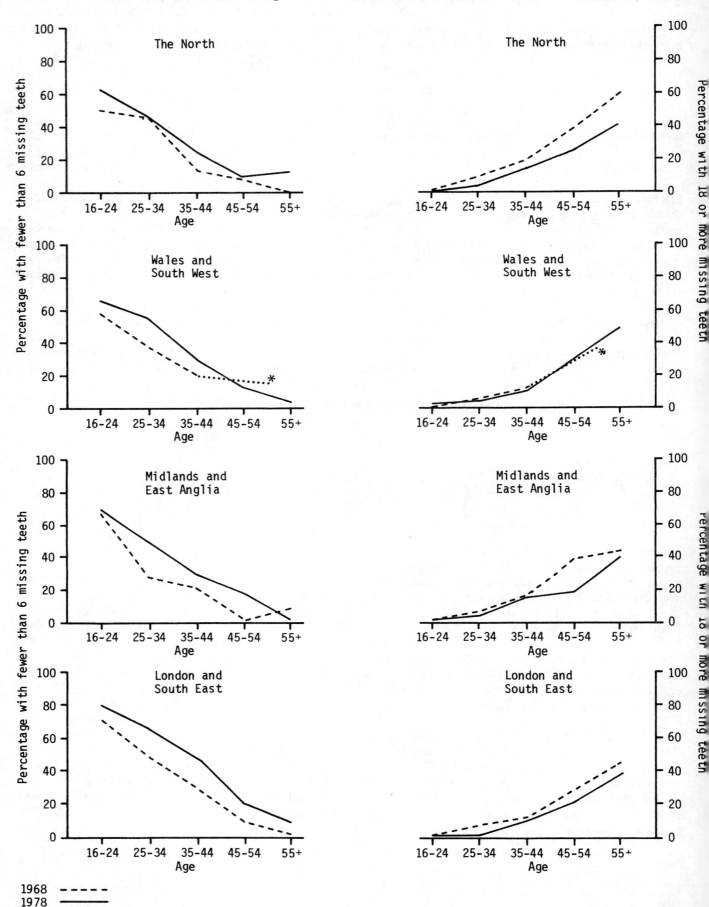

1968 ------
1978 ———

*Because of small base sizes, the two age groups have been amalgamated

regions had achieved by 1978 and yet still further improvement had been made.

In terms of the proportion of people with large numbers of teeth missing, the desirable situation is for the 1978 figures to be lower than those in 1968. This was consistently the case for people of all ages in the North and in London and the South East but there was no difference for younger dentate adults in the other regions.

6.4 Sound and untreated teeth

It might at first glance seem perfectly reasonable to study the variation in the number of sound and untreated teeth in the community and use this as an indicator of dental disease. However, for the reasons discussed in Section 6.2, if filled teeth, decayed teeth and missing teeth are taken together to imply a disease level, which is the same as taking sound, untreated teeth as an indicator of lack of disease, then it is not uncommon to present results which appear to suggest that people who seek dental care have more disease than people who do not.

Any detailed analysis of disease levels on this basis are therefore very undesirable as they contain artefacts related both to the survey method and the provision of dental treatment. It is, however, reasonable to examine the data to establish one basic fact of importance, that is that dental decay in adults is more or less universal. Although it is true that estimating the number of teeth that have at some time suffered from decay is not possible, it is feasible to identify the proportion of mouths that appear to have had very little treatment indeed and no sign of decay. In 1968 an analysis of the examination charts was carried out to identify how many people had no evidence of disease at all. Only 7 people in the whole sample were apparently totally free from decay experience. We have not carried out the detailed investigation to replicate this analysis but it is possible to look at the numbers of people who have a large number of sound and untreated teeth and check whether in 1978 it is still true to say that only a tiny minority of people escape from the problems of dental decay. In 1968 1.5% of dentate people had 27 or more sound and untreated teeth. In 1978 the comparable figure was 2.9%. So it is still the case that practically everyone (97% of dentate adults) had evidence of some past or present dental disease. Consequently, at present it would seem that an investment in restorative work is the best insurance for a lifelong reliance on natural teeth.

6.5 Filled (otherwise sound) teeth

We saw in Table 6.1 that the average number of filled teeth for dentate adults had risen by one tooth over the ten year period between the surveys. Table 6.4 shows the average number of filled (otherwise sound) teeth for men and women separately and according to age. For both sexes and for all age groups except the youngest, the average number of filled (otherwise sound) teeth had increased. The decrease among the 16 to 24 year olds was not statistically significant.

Assuming that edentulousness was not making an impact on the figures for people aged less than 45 we can see that the increase in the average number of filled (otherwise sound) teeth for people aged 25 or more was due not particularly to higher treatment levels in the last ten years, but rather to a difference in the treatment experience of different age cohorts. For example, dentate adults aged 25 to 34 in 1968 had on average 8.6 filled teeth, while dentate adults aged 35 to 44 at that time had 6.7 filled teeth. In 1978 we find that dentate adults now aged 35 to 44, that is, (except for people having become edentulous) the dentate adults aged 25 to 34 ten years earlier, have, on average, 8.6 filled (otherwise sound) teeth.

In other words, adults who were still dentate in 1978 were maintaining much the same situation with respect to fillings as they had ten years previously. Only for the dentate adults aged 25 to 34 in 1978 did there appear to be an additional increase in restorative treatment during the past ten years. The figures suggest that restorative treatment for the age group 16 to 24 and earlier is of considerable consequence for future dental conditions.

The increase in the average number of filled (otherwise sound) teeth found among dentate adults was also to be seen when the regions were examined. The relationship between the regions therefore remained much the same as it was in 1968.

Since so few people escape from problems of dental decay, the provision of restorative treatment, the most common form of which is fillings, plays a very important part in enabling people to retain their natural teeth. Contrary to initial expectations therefore, it might be argued that it is a disadvantage for future dental health to find a high proportion of people who currently have no fillings. Until the amount of decay people experience can be radically reduced, restorative work is essential. It is particularly interesting, therefore, to look at the extremes of the distributions of the number of filled (otherwise sound) teeth to see whether there have been any changes in the proportion of dentate adults who have no filled

Table 6.4 Mean number of filled (otherwise sound) teeth among dentate people in different age groups in 1968 and 1978

Age	Male		Female		Both sexes	
	1968	1978	1968	1978	1968	1978
16-24	7.8 *171*	7.2 *283*	8.6 *200*	8.1 *284*	8.2 *371*	7.7 *567*
25-34	7.2 *226*	8.3 *271*	10.0 *219*	10.5 *370*	8.6 *445*	9.6 *641*
35-44	6.2 *221*	8.1 *277*	7.2 *175*	9.2 *251*	6.7 *396*	8.6 *528*
45-54	5.2 *124*	6.6 *210*	4.8 *133*	7.1 *173*	5.0 *257*	6.8 *383*
55 and over	3.1 *116*	4.1 *203*	4.0 *109*	5.2 *164*	3.5 *225*	4.6 *367*
All ages	6.2 *858*	7.0 *1244*	7.5 *836*	8.5 *1242*	6.8 *1694*	7.8 *2486*

Figure 6.2 **Proportion of dentate adults in different age groups with no filled (otherwise sound) teeth and of those with 12 or more filled (otherwise sound) teeth**

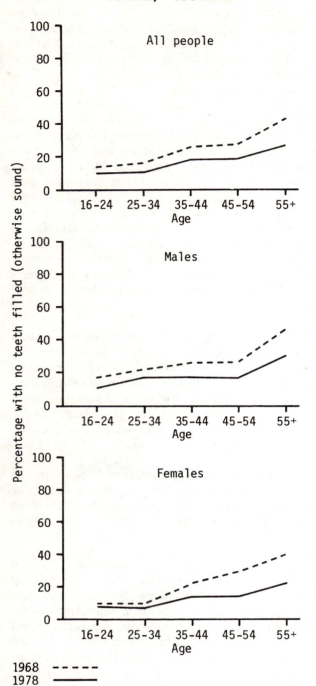

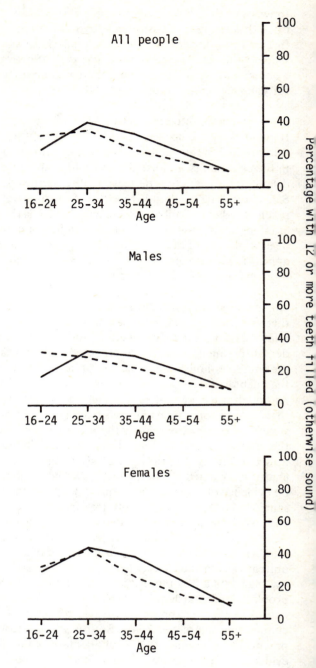

1968 ----
1978 ——

(otherwise sound) teeth and the proportion who have 12 or more teeth of this kind.

Figure 6.2 shows the results for different age groups and sexes. In overall terms the proportion of dentate adults who had no filled teeth fell from 23% in 1968 to 14% in 1978*. This reduction was evident among all age groups and for both men and women.

The overall figures for the proportion of dentate adults who had 12 or more filled (otherwise sound) teeth had remained fairly constant over the last ten years (25% in

---

* These figures together with the complete distributions will be found at the end of this chapter.

Table 6.5 Mean number of filled (otherwise sound) teeth among dentate people in different regions in 1968 and 1978

Regions	1968		1978	
The North	5.6	436	6.6	620
Wales & the South West	7.0	213	8.2	434
Midlands & East Anglia	6.0	373	7.0	590
London & the South East	8.0	672	8.9	842
England & Wales	6.8	1694	7.8	2486

1968 compared to 27% in 1978). There was some variation with age however. The youngest age group, especially the males, had a smaller proportion of people with a large number of filled teeth. In the middle age ranges, on the other hand, a higher proportion of both men and women had evidence of extensive restorative treatment in 1978.

Although for all age groups there had been a reduction in the proportion of dentate adults who had no filled (otherwise sound) teeth and although there was a reduction in all regions, there still remained a fairly large difference in the levels found in the North and in London and the South East.

Figure 6.3 shows that restorative dentistry was still more universal in the South and that extensive restorative treatment was still more evident there.

The level of restorative treatment obtained is, of course, closely related to a person's motivation and behaviour and the 1968 report showed how different the dental treatment patterns were for those people who attended the dentist for a regular check-up and those who only went to the dentist when they were having trouble with their teeth.

Attendance pattern is clearly such a fundamentally important variable that it is of interest in its own right and later in Chapter 8 results are presented showing the changes that have taken place. At this point, however, dental attendance pattern is of interest in terms of its relationship with restorative dentistry.

We described earlier why it is that not having any fillings is not the asset it might, on first reflection, be thought to be, since, given the almost universal nature of dental disease, it is usually an indicator of a lack of required treatment than of lack of disease. Figure 6.4 shows the proportion of dentate adults with no filled (otherwise sound) teeth according to age and dental attendance pattern*. It also shows the proportion of dentate adults with 12 or more filled teeth. The diagrams clearly bear out the paradox described above for virtually no one who is a regular attender had no fillings, and it is also the case that very few of those who only attend when they have trouble with their teeth have 12 or more which were filled (otherwise sound). It is encouraging for the future, however, that a considerable reduction has taken place among the worst attendance group in the proportion who had no teeth which were filled (otherwise sound).

We have seen in Figure 6.3 that there were considerable differences in the level of restorative treatment in the North and in London and the South East, although the

* As was the case in 1968, the 1978 survey established dental attendance pattern from the interview by asking informants if they went to the dentist for a regular check-up, an occasional check-up or only when they were having trouble with their teeth. For the analysis of the condition of the natural teeth only the two main groups, the first and last of the three, are used.

Figure 6.3   Proportion of dentate adults in different age groups and regions with no filled (otherwise sound) teeth and of those with 12 or more filled (otherwise sound) teeth

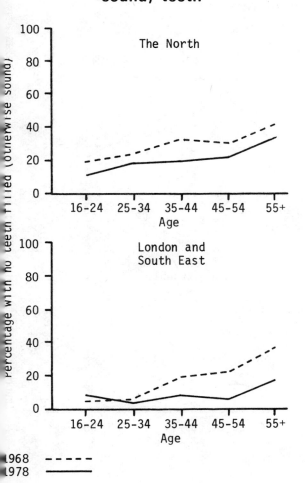
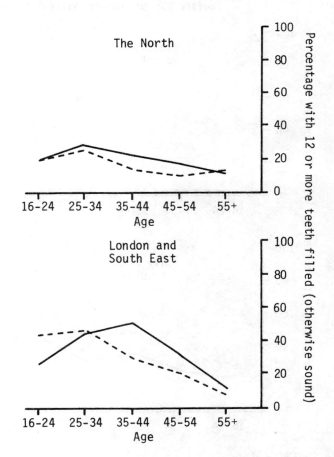

1968 - - - - -
1978 ————

23

situation had improved over ten years. Since dental attendance is so highly correlated with the kind of treatment received, we examine whether the regional variation was accounted for by a regional difference in attendance pattern. It is not possible with the numbers of variables involved to provide results in full detail but we show the comparisons for the relevant sub-groups in which variation would be found if attendance pattern were the explanation for regional variation.

In the North the proportion of regular attenders who had 12 or more filled (otherwise sound) teeth had risen marginally over ten years, while the proportion for similar people in London and the South East had actually decreased, thus reducing the regional variation.

For people who only attend when they have trouble with their teeth, a greater proportion had evidence of some restorative treatment in 1978 whichever region they were from. Once again, London and the South East was the region which started off from a better position and also appeared to make most progress. This progress was not only evident in terms of the proportion of those who only go to the dentist with trouble who had some fillings, but also in the proportion who had 12 or more filled (otherwise sound) teeth. The figures thus show that the regional improvements with respect to the indicators of restorative treatment had been achieved among people who do not exhibit high dental motivation.

6.6 Decayed teeth
In the survey dental examination, decayed teeth were recorded in three different categories, filled and decayed, decayed not previously treated but restorable, and not

Table 6.6 The proportion of filled (otherwise sound) teeth among dentate adults from different regions and with differing attendance patterns

Dentate adults who go to the dentist for a regular check-up

	The North		London & the South East	
	1968	1978	1968	1978
Proportion with 12 or more filled (otherwise sound) teeth	39% 160	41% 258	53% 297	48% 394

Dentate adults who only go to the dentist when they are having trouble

	The North		London & the South East	
	1968	1978	1968	1978
Proportion with no filled (otherwise sound) teeth	48% 230	38% 282	31% 296	16% 302
Proportion with 12 or more filled (otherwise sound) teeth	4% 230	4% 282	8% 296	19% 302

Figure 6.4 Proportion of dentate adults of different attendance patterns and in different age groups with no filled (otherwise sound) teeth and of those with 12 or more filled (otherwise sound) teeth

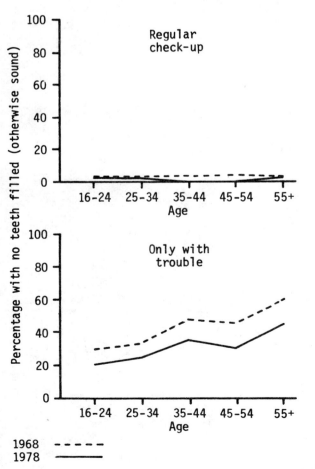

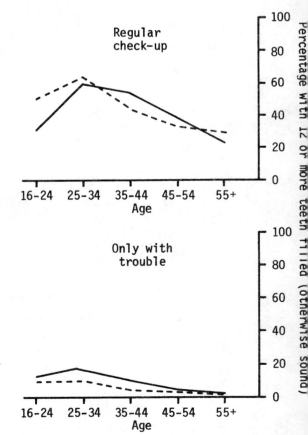

1968 - - - - -
1978 ————

restorable. Included in the first category are unsound fillings that need replacement.

The 1978 survey showed that among dentate adults an average of 1.9 teeth were found to be decayed compared with 2.2 in 1968. This difference was not statistically significant and so the survey results show no change in the average level of decay, as measured by the survey dental examination, over the last ten years.

Again it is of interest to look at indicators that reflect the number of teeth that are involved with particular conditions. When looking at decayed teeth the indicator used is the proportion of people with some decayed teeth. In 1968, 64% of dentate people had some decay, in 1978 this proportion had fallen slightly but there were still 59% of dentate people recorded as having some decay.

Figure 6.5 shows that this small difference was found only for people aged less than 45. Analysis for the two sexes showed similar very small levels of change which resulted in a greater proportion of men than of women having active decay, as we had found in 1968.

Figure 6.5 also shows the situation with respect to active decay in the North and London and the South East and again shows only slight change, although there was an unexpected increase in the proportion of people with some teeth classified as decayed among those aged 45 or more in London and the South East.

Of all the variables that one would expect to be related to active decay, attendance pattern must, of course, be extremely relevant. The last part of Figure 6.5 shows, for dentate adults who go for a regular check-up and for those who go only when they are having trouble with their teeth, the proportion who were found to have some decay.

As in 1968, nearly half the regular attenders in 1978 were found to have one or more teeth classified as decayed. It must be remembered here that unsound fillings are included in this category as they represent a treatment need. In fact among the regular attenders in 1978 the average number of decayed teeth was 1.1 and this comprised 0.8 decayed and filled, 0.3 decayed but restorable and no unrestorable teeth. Thus the major treatment need for regular attenders involved teeth that had already been restored.

As far as those people who only go to the dentist when they are having trouble with their teeth were concerned, the proportion with some decay was, of course, high compared with regular attenders. However, among the younger age groups the proportion who had some decay was lower in 1978 than it had been in 1968. As with the regular attenders, it is of interest to look at the contribution of the different categories of decay recorded. Overall, people who only go to the dentist when they had trouble with their teeth had, in 1978, 2.9 teeth classified as decayed. This comprised 0.7 that were filled and decayed, 1.5 that were decayed but restorable and 0.7 that were unrestorable. So, not only did these people have a higher average number of decayed teeth than regular dental attenders (2.9 compared with 1.1) but the kind of decay recorded was also of a more serious nature in terms of their dental prognosis and this was as true in 1978 as it had been in 1968.

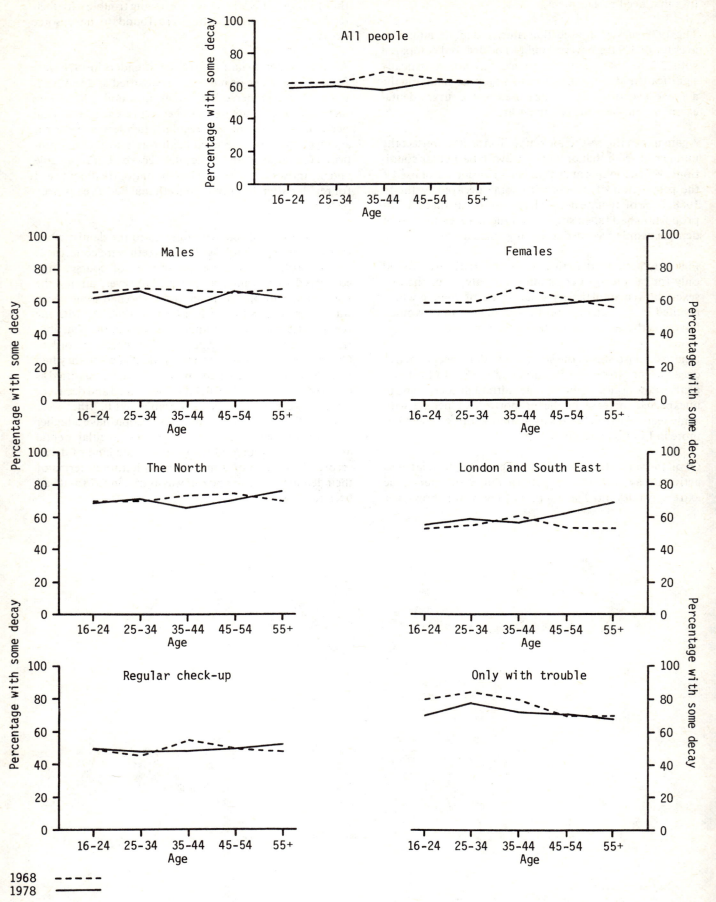

1968 - - - - -
1978 ———

Table 6A.1 Distribution of numbers of missing teeth among dentate adults in different age groups by sex

No. of missing teeth	Age											
	16-24		25-34		35-44		45-54		55 and over		All ages	
	1968	1978	1968	1978	1968	1978	1968	1978	1968	1978	1968	1978
	Males											
	%	%	%	%	%	%	%	%	%	%	%	%
0	2	5	3	7	2	3	1	1	1	1	2	3
1-5	65	67	38	49	22	33	9	15	3	6	31	37
6-11	28	25	43	35	44	44	32	36	17	25	35	33
12-17	4	2	10	5	19	11	30	27	33	25	17	13
18 or more	1	1	6	4	13	9	28	21	46	43	15	14
Total	100	100	100	100	100	100	100	100	100	100	100	100
Mean	4.9	4.7	7.3	5.9	10.0	8.2	13.7	12.0	17.1	16.3	9.8	8.9
Base	*171*	*283*	*226*	*271*	*221*	*277*	*124*	*210*	*116*	*203*	*858*	*1244*
	Females											
	%	%	%	%	%	%	%	%	%	%	%	%
0	4	5	3	4	—	1	1	—	—	1	2	3
1-5	55	65	40	50	21	30	7	13	5	6	30	38
6-11	38	28	39	36	43	43	29	36	16	20	35	34
12-17	2	1	11	8	19	11	25	27	30	35	15	13
18 or more	1	1	7	2	17	15	38	24	49	38	18	12
Total	100	100	100	100	100	100	100	100	100	100	100	100
Mean	5.4	4.7	7.6	6.2	11.0	9.4	15.2	12.7	17.5	15.7	10.3	8.7
Base	*200*	*284*	*219*	*370*	*175*	*251*	*133*	*173*	*109*	*164*	*836*	*1242*
	Both sexes											
	%	%	%	%	%	%	%	%	%	%	%	%
0	3	5	3	5	1	2	1	—	—	1	2	3
1-5	60	66	39	50	22	32	8	14	4	6	30	38
6-11	33	27	41	35	44	43	30	36	17	23	35	33
12-17	3	1	10	7	19	11	27	27	32	29	16	13
18 or more	1	1	7	3	14	12	34	23	47	41	17	13
Total	100	100	100	100	100	100	100	100	100	100	100	100
Mean	5.2	4.7	7.5	6.0	10.5	8.8	14.5	12.3	17.3	16.0	10.1	8.8
Base	*371*	*567*	*445*	*641*	*396*	*528*	*257*	*383*	*225*	*367*	*1694*	*2486*

Table 6A.2 **Distribution of numbers of missing teeth among dentate adults in different age groups by region**

No. of missing teeth	Age 16-24 1968	1978	25-34 1968	1978	35-44 1968	1978	45-54 1968	1978	55 and over 1968	1978	All ages 1968	1978
	The North											
	%	%	%	%	%	%	%	%	%	%	%	%
0	3	2	4	4	—	2	—	—	—	—	2	2
1-5	48	62	42	42	12	21	7	8	—	10	27	34
6-11	45	33	38	43	47	50	22	43	21	16	38	39
12-17	3	3	9	8	22	12	31	25	20	33	15	13
18 or more	1	—	7	3	19	15	40	24	59	41	18	12
Total	100	100	100	100	100	100	100	100	100	100	100	100
Mean	5.8	5.0	7.3	6.7	11.6	10.0	16.0	13.0	18.2	16.5	10.3	9.0
Base	*119*	*148*	*107*	*176*	*101*	*130*	*58*	*98*	*51*	*68*	*436*	*620*
	Wales and the South West											
	%	%	%	%	%	%	%	%	%	%	%	%
0	—	3	3	2	2	1	3	—	—	—	2	2
1-5	58	63	35	52	19	28	13	12	(3)	3	30	35
6-11	38	30	47	34	48	43	25	31	(4)	21	39	35
12-17	4	2	10	8	21	20	31	29	(7)	28	17	15
18 or more	—	2	5	4	10	8	28	28	(8)	48	12	15
Total	100	100	100	100	100	100	100	100		100	100	100
Mean	5.2	5.3	7.7	6.3	10.1	8.9	13.8	13.4	*	17.9	9.5	9.5
Base	*45*	*95*	*62*	*110*	*52*	*95*	*32*	*71*	*(22)*	*63*	*213*	*434*
	Midlands and East Anglia											
	%	%	%	%	%	%	%	%	%	%	%	%
0	2	7	2	4	—	5	—	—	—	—	1	4
1-5	65	63	25	47	22	26	2	15	8	1	28	34
6-11	29	28	54	38	39	48	29	38	14	28	36	36
12-17	3	1	13	7	23	6	30	29	34	31	18	13
18 or more	1	1	6	4	16	15	39	18	44	40	17	13
Total	100	100	100	100	100	100	100	100	100	100	100	100
Mean	5.1	4.6	8.3	6.2	11.2	9.0	15.8	11.8	16.7	15.8	10.4	8.7
Base	*88*	*137*	*98*	*147*	*86*	*128*	*51*	*85*	*50*	*92*	*373*	*590*
	London and the South East											
	%	%	%	%	%	%	%	%	%	%	%	%
0	5	8	3	8	2	—	1	1	1	1	2	4
1-5	68	72	46	58	28	46	10	19	2	9	33	44
6-11	24	19	35	29	43	36	37	33	16	24	32	28
12-17	2	—	9	4	15	9	23	26	36	28	16	12
18 or more	1	1	7	1	12	9	29	21	45	38	17	12
Total	100	100	100	100	100	100	100	100	100	100	100	100
Mean	4.7	4.2	7.1	5.2	9.4	7.7	13.4	11.6	17.5	15.2	9.9	8.2
Base	*119*	*187*	*178*	*208*	*157*	*175*	*116*	*129*	*102*	*143*	*672*	*842*

* *Percentages and means are not given for bases of less than 30.*

Table 6A.3 Distribution of numbers of missing teeth among dentate adults in different age groups by dental attendance pattern

No. of missing teeth	Age											
	16-24		25-34		35-44		45-54		55 and over		All ages	
	1968	1978	1968	1978	1968	1978	1968	1978	1968	1978	1968	1978
	\multicolumn{12}{l}{People who go to the dentist for regular check-ups}											
	%	%	%	%	%	%	%	%	%	%	%	%
0	4	4	1	5	2	1	1	1	—	1	2	3
1-5	63	67	51	54	29	38	13	18	8	10	40	43
6-11	29	26	41	34	44	47	42	45	27	34	38	37
12-17	3	2	5	5	18	9	25	22	43	27	13	10
18 or more	1	1	2	2	7	5	19	14	22	28	7	7
Total	100	100	100	100	100	100	100	100	100	100	100	100
Mean	4.9	4.8	6.0	5.6	8.6	7.4	11.8	10.5	13.2	13.4	7.8	7.4
Base	169	263	197	320	164	264	90	171	60	130	680	1148
	\multicolumn{12}{l}{People who only go to the dentist when they have trouble with their teeth}											
	%	%	%	%	%	%	%	%	%	%	%	%
0	2	6	3	5	—	2	1	—	—	—	1	3
1-5	50	65	25	44	15	24	6	11	1	2	20	30
6-11	43	27	43	39	41	42	22	26	14	18	34	31
12-17	4	1	17	7	22	15	28	31	24	30	19	16
18 or more	1	1	12	5	22	17	43	32	61	50	26	20
Total	100	100	100	100	100	100	100	100	100	100	100	100
Mean	5.8	4.7	9.3	6.7	12.3	10.2	16.2	14.2	19.3	18.0	12.4	10.6
Base	143	197	191	218	195	197	144	173	144	197	817	983

Table 6A.4 Distribution of numbers of sound teeth among dentate adults in different age groups by sex

No. of sound teeth	Age											
	16-24		25-34		35-44		45-54		55 and over		All ages	
	1968	1978	1968	1978	1968	1978	1968	1978	1968	1978	1968	1978
	\multicolumn{12}{l}{Males}											
	%	%	%	%	%	%	%	%	%	%	%	%
0	—	—	—	1	—	—	2	1	5	5	1	1
1-5	2	2	6	7	10	7	16	11	29	27	11	10
6-11	12	13	26	19	30	35	38	48	34	34	27	28
12-17	37	28	35	39	39	33	32	28	20	23	34	31
18 or more	49	57	33	34	21	25	12	12	12	11	27	30
Total	100	100	100	100	100	100	100	100	100	100	100	100
Mean	16.7	17.8	14.7	15.0	13.0	13.4	10.6	11.0	9.2	9.1	13.3	13.6
Base	171	283	226	271	221	277	124	210	116	203	858	1244
	\multicolumn{12}{l}{Females}											
	%	%	%	%	%	%	%	%	%	%	%	%
0	—	—	1	1	2	1	2	2	3	3	1	1
1-5	1	2	6	4	9	10	14	14	28	22	9	9
6-11	17	14	37	32	40	46	52	49	42	45	36	35
12-17	42	35	44	40	32	29	24	25	19	21	35	32
18 or more	40	49	12	23	17	14	8	10	8	9	19	23
Total	100	100	100	100	100	100	100	100	100	100	100	100
Mean	16.1	17.3	12.5	13.5	11.9	11.4	10.0	10.1	8.6	9.2	12.3	12.9
Base	200	284	219	370	175	251	133	173	109	164	836	1242
	\multicolumn{12}{l}{Both sexes}											
	%	%	%	%	%	%	%	%	%	%	%	%
0	—	—	—	1	1	—	2	2	4	4	1	1
1-5	2	2	6	6	9	9	15	12	28	25	10	9
6-11	15	14	31	26	35	40	45	49	38	38	31	32
12-17	39	31	40	39	36	31	28	26	20	22	35	31
18 or more	44	53	23	28	19	20	10	11	10	11	23	27
Total	100	100	100	100	100	100	100	100	100	100	100	100
Mean	16.4	17.5	13.6	14.1	12.5	12.5	10.3	10.6	8.9	9.1	12.8	13.2
Base	371	567	445	641	396	528	257	383	225	367	1694	2486

Table 6A.5 Distribution of numbers of sound teeth among dentate adults in different age groups by region

No. of sound teeth	Age											
	16-24		25-34		35-44		45-54		55 and over		All ages	
	1968	1978	1968	1978	1968	1978	1968	1978	1968	1978	1968	1978
The North	%	%	%	%	%	%	%	%	%	%	%	%
0	—	—	1	—	1	—	3	2	2	4	1	1
1-5	2	3	7	4	9	8	17	12	31	33	10	9
6-11	13	13	24	26	39	36	45	48	49	37	30	30
12-17	36	37	36	39	29	38	30	30	12	16	31	34
18 or more	49	47	32	31	22	18	5	8	6	10	28	26
Total	100	100	100	100	100	100	100	100	100	100	100	100
Mean	16.9	16.5	14.9	14.9	12.3	12.4	9.4	10.1	8.1	8.3	13.3	13.3
Base	*119*	*148*	*107*	*176*	*101*	*130*	*58*	*98*	*51*	*68*	*436*	*620*
Wales and the South West	%	%	%	%	%	%	%	%	%	%	%	%
0	—	—	—	2	—	2	3	1	(1)	4	1	2
1-5	—	3	3	8	14	5	19	13	(4)	30	9	10
6-11	20	17	32	30	25	45	28	49	(8)	39	28	35
12-17	38	34	44	35	48	29	41	28	(5)	20	41	30
18 or more	42	46	21	25	13	19	9	9	(4)	7	21	23
Total	100	100	100	100	100	100	100	100		100	100	100
Mean	16.2	17.0	13.2	13.3	12.1	12.1	10.4	10.7	*	8.5	12.8	12.7
Base	*45*	*94*	*62*	*110*	*52*	*95*	*32*	*71*	*(22)*	*63*	*213*	*434*
Midlands and East Anglia	%	%	%	%	%	%	%	%	%	%	%	%
0	—	—	—	1	1	—	2	1	4	2	1	1
1-5	—	1	6	6	11	5	22	11	22	16	10	7
6-11	11	11	29	24	30	38	31	47	42	38	27	29
12-17	41	30	41	41	37	28	29	21	18	33	35	32
18 or more	48	58	24	28	21	29	16	20	14	11	27	31
Total	100	100	100	100	100	100	100	100	100	100	100	100
Mean	17.1	18.6	14.1	14.2	12.8	14.2	10.5	11.8	10.0	10.4	13.4	14.3
Base	*88*	*137*	*98*	*147*	*86*	*128*	*51*	*85*	*50*	*92*	*373*	*590*
London and the South East	%	%	%	%	%	%	%	%	%	%	%	%
0	—	—	1	2	1	1	1	3	5	6	1	2
1-5	2	2	6	5	8	13	10	13	32	24	10	11
6-11	18	14	36	27	36	41	56	49	30	41	36	33
12-17	43	27	40	40	36	30	23	26	24	19	34	29
18 or more	37	57	17	26	19	15	10	9	9	10	19	25
Total	100	100	100	100	100	100	100	100	100	100	100	100
Mean	15.5	17.8	12.7	13.9	12.6	11.4	10.6	10.1	8.7	8.9	12.2	12.8
Base	*119*	*187*	*178*	*208*	*157*	*175*	*116*	*129*	*102*	*143*	*672*	*842*

* Percentages and means are not given for bases of less than 30.

Table 6A.6 Distribution of numbers of sound teeth among dentate adults in different age groups by dental attendance pattern

No. of sound teeth	Age											
	16-24		25-34		35-44		45-54		55 and over		All ages	
	1968	1978	1968	1978	1968	1978	1968	1978	1968	1978	1968	1978
People who go to the dentist for regular check-ups	%	%	%	%	%	%	%	%	%	%	%	%
0	—	—	—	1	1	—	2	1	5	5	1	1
1-5	2	1	5	7	9	9	13	15	22	19	8	9
6-11	25	19	39	33	44	48	46	50	45	47	38	37
12-17	46	38	45	42	38	32	37	28	23	24	40	35
18 or more	27	42	11	17	8	11	2	6	5	5	13	18
Total	100	100	100	100	100	100	100	100	100	100	100	100
Mean	14.3	16.1	12.3	12.4	11.1	11.0	9.8	10.0	8.8	8.9	11.8	12.2
Base	*169*	*263*	*197*	*320*	*164*	*264*	*90*	*171*	*60*	*130*	*680*	*1148*
People who only go to the dentist when they have trouble with their teeth	%	%	%	%	%	%	%	%	%	%	%	%
0	—	—	—	1	1	1	2	3	4	4	1	2
1-5	1	3	8	4	10	9	16	11	32	30	13	11
6-11	3	9	25	19	26	28	42	43	35	33	26	26
12-17	34	22	32	35	32	31	25	26	19	22	29	28
18 or more	62	66	35	41	31	31	15	17	10	11	31	33
Total	100	100	100	100	100	100	100	100	100	100	100	100
Mean	18.6	19.0	14.7	16.1	13.7	14.3	10.7	11.3	8.6	9.0	13.3	14.1
Base	*143*	*197*	*191*	*218*	*195*	*197*	*144*	*173*	*144*	*197*	*817*	*983*

Table 6A.7 Distribution of numbers of teeth which were filled (otherwise sound) among dentate adults in different age groups by sex

No. of teeth filled (otherwise sound)	Age											
	16-24		25-34		35-44		45-54		55 and over		All ages	
	1968	1978	1968	1978	1968	1978	1968	1978	1968	1978	1968	1978
	Males											
	%	%	%	%	%	%	%	%	%	%	%	%
0	17	11	22	16	26	16	25	15	46	29	26	17
1-5	20	28	25	20	24	19	34	31	29	38	26	26
6-11	31	44	25	32	28	35	28	34	17	25	26	35
12 or more	32	17	28	32	22	30	13	20	8	8	22	22
Total	100	100	100	100	100	100	100	100	100	100	100	100
Mean	7.8	7.2	7.2	8.3	6.2	8.1	5.2	6.6	3.1	4.1	6.2	7.0
Base	*171*	*283*	*226*	*271*	*221*	*277*	*124*	*210*	*116*	*203*	*858*	*1244*
	Females											
	%	%	%	%	%	%	%	%	%	%	%	%
0	10	8	10	6	22	14	29	15	41	22	20	11
1-5	21	25	12	12	21	16	37	26	28	37	22	21
6-11	37	39	34	37	32	31	18	37	20	31	30	36
12 or more	32	28	44	45	25	39	16	22	11	10	28	32
Total	100	100	100	100	100	100	100	100	100	100	100	100
Mean	8.6	8.1	10.0	10.5	7.2	9.2	4.8	7.1	4.0	5.2	7.5	8.5
Base	*200*	*284*	*219*	*370*	*175*	*251*	*133*	*173*	*109*	*164*	*836*	*1242*
	Both sexes											
	%	%	%	%	%	%	%	%	%	%	%	%
0	14	9	16	10	24	15	27	15	43	26	23	14
1-5	20	27	19	15	23	18	35	29	29	38	24	24
6-11	34	41	29	35	29	33	23	35	19	27	28	35
12 or more	32	23	36	40	24	34	15	21	9	9	25	27
Total	100	100	100	100	100	100	100	100	100	100	100	100
Mean	8.2	7.7	8.6	9.6	6.7	8.6	5.0	6.8	3.5	4.6	6.8	7.8
Base	*371*	*567*	*445*	*641*	*396*	*528*	*257*	*383*	*225*	*367*	*1694*	*2486*

Table 6A.8 Distribution of numbers of teeth which were filled (otherwise sound) among dentate adults in different age groups by region

No. of teeth filled (otherwise sound)	Age											
	16-24		25-34		35-44		45-54		55 and over		All ages	
	1968	1978	1968	1978	1968	1978	1968	1978	1968	1978	1968	1978
The North												
	%	%	%	%	%	%	%	%	%	%	%	%
0	19	9	24	19	32	20	29	22	43	33	28	19
1-5	26	30	20	22	25	24	42	29	31	38	27	27
6-11	35	41	30	31	28	34	19	33	14	19	27	33
12 or more	20	20	26	28	15	22	10	16	12	10	18	21
Total	100	100	100	100	100	100	100	100	100	100	100	100
Mean	6.5	7.3	6.9	7.3	5.2	7.0	4.2	5.8	3.3	4.1	5.6	6.6
Base	*119*	*148*	*107*	*176*	*101*	*130*	*58*	*98*	*51*	*68*	*436*	*620*
Wales and the South West												
	%	%	%	%	%	%	%	%	%	%	%	%
0	9	8	26	7	23	12	28	13	(11)	29	24	12
1-5	29	23	16	13	19	15	31	35	(4)	33	22	23
6-11	27	46	21	38	29	35	25	34	(5)	30	25	37
12 or more	35	23	37	42	29	38	16	18	(2)	8	29	28
Total	100	100	100	100	100	100	100	100	100	100	100	100
Mean	8.2	8.2	7.9	10.8	7.1	9.4	5.3	6.3	(22)	4.1	7.0	8.2
Base	*45*	*94*	*62*	*110*	*52*	*95*	*32*	*71*	*(22)*	*63*	*213*	*434*
Midlands and East Anglia												
	%	%	%	%	%	%	%	%	%	%	%	%
0	22	13	21	11	23	23	37	21	54	36	28	20
1-5	15	28	24	14	28	24	39	26	22	35	24	24
6-11	33	36	34	33	27	30	16	34	12	25	27	32
12 or more	30	23	21	42	22	23	8	19	12	4	21	24
Total	100	100	100	100	100	100	100	100	100	100	100	100
Mean	7.8	7.1	6.9	9.7	6.0	6.8	3.4	6.4	3.6	3.7	6.0	7.0
Base	*88*	*137*	*98*	*147*	*86*	*128*	*51*	*85*	*50*	*92*	*373*	*590*
London and the South East												
	%	%	%	%	%	%	%	%	%	%	%	%
0	4	7	5	3	19	7	22	5	36	15	16	7
1-5	15	25	17	12	20	9	32	28	33	42	23	22
6-11	38	43	29	38	33	35	27	38	24	32	30	37
12 or more	43	25	49	47	28	49	19	29	7	11	31	34
Total	100	100	100	100	100	100	100	100	100	100	100	100
Mean	10.2	8.1	10.7	10.8	7.8	10.8	5.9	8.0	3.6	5.6	8.0	8.9
Base	*119*	*187*	*178*	*208*	*157*	*175*	*116*	*129*	*102*	*143*	*672*	*842*

* *Percentages and means are not given for bases of less than 30.*

Table 6A.9 Distribution of numbers of teeth which are filled (otherwise sound) among dentate adults by attendance pattern in different age groups

No. of missing teeth	Age											
	16-24		25-34		35-44		45-54		55 and over		All ages	
	1968	1978	1968	1978	1968	1978	1968	1978	1968	1978	1968	1978
	People who go to the dentist for regular check-ups											
	%	%	%	%	%	%	%	%	%	%	%	%
0	1	1	1	1	2	—	3	—	2	1	2	1
1-5	8	18	6	5	13	7	23	17	27	30	12	13
6-11	40	49	29	36	41	39	40	45	43	47	37	42
12 or more	51	32	64	58	44	54	34	38	28	22	49	44
Total	100	100	100	100	100	100	100	100	100	100	100	100
Mean	11.5	9.6	12.7	12.4	10.8	12.1	9.0	9.9	8.7	8.2	11.1	10.8
Base	*169*	*263*	*197*	*320*	*164*	*264*	*90*	*171*	*60*	*130*	*680*	*1148*
	People who only go to the dentist when they have trouble with their teeth											
	%	%	%	%	%	%	%	%	%	%	%	%
0	29	20	33	24	47	36	45	31	61	44	43	31
1-5	35	39	33	31	32	27	41	42	30	41	34	36
6-11	28	29	25	28	17	27	11	23	8	13	18	24
12 or more	8	12	9	17	4	10	3	4	1	2	5	9
Total	100	100	100	100	100	100	100	100	100	100	100	100
Mean	4.2	5.3	4.4	5.7	2.8	4.5	2.2	3.5	1.3	2.2	3.0	4.3
Base	*143*	*197*	*191*	*218*	*195*	*197*	*144*	*173*	*144*	*197*	*817*	*983*

Table 6A.10 Distribution of numbers of decayed teeth among dentate adults in different age groups by sex

No. of decayed teeth	Age											
	16-24		25-34		35-44		45-54		55 and over		All ages	
	1968	1978	1968	1978	1968	1978	1968	1978	1968	1978	1968	1978
	Males											
	%	%	%	%	%	%	%	%	%	%	%	%
0	34	37	32	33	33	43	35	34	33	37	33	37
1-5	52	51	52	52	53	48	54	57	52	54	53	52
6 or more	14	12	16	15	14	9	11	9	15	9	14	11
Total	100	100	100	100	100	100	100	100	100	100	100	100
Mean	2.5	2.2	2.8	2.5	2.6	1.9	2.4	2.0	2.5	2.2	2.6	2.2
Base	*171*	*283*	*226*	*271*	*221*	*277*	*124*	*210*	*116*	*203*	*858*	*1244*
	Females											
	%	%	%	%	%	%	%	%	%	%	%	%
0	42	47	42	46	33	43	38	41	44	39	40	44
1-5	49	45	49	48	62	50	52	52	46	52	52	49
6 or more	9	8	9	6	5	7	10	7	10	9	8	7
Total	100	100	100	100	100	100	100	100	100	100	100	100
Mean	1.8	1.7	1.9	1.5	1.7	1.6	1.9	1.7	2.0	1.7	1.8	1.6
Base	*200*	*284*	*219*	*370*	*175*	*251*	*133*	*173*	*109*	*164*	*836*	*1242*
	Both sexes											
	%	%	%	%	%	%	%	%	%	%	%	%
0	38	42	37	40	33	43	36	37	38	38	36	41
1-5	50	48	51	50	57	49	53	55	49	53	52	50
6 or more	12	10	12	10	10	8	11	8	13	9	12	9
Total	100	100	100	100	100	100	100	100	100	100	100	100
Mean	2.1	2.0	2.3	1.9	2.2	1.8	2.2	1.9	2.2	2.0	2.2	1.9
Base	*371*	*567*	*445*	*641*	*396*	*528*	*257*	*383*	*225*	*367*	*1694*	*2486*

Table 6A.11 Distribution of numbers of decayed teeth among dentate adults in different age groups by region

No. of decayed teeth	Age											
	16-24		25-34		35-44		45-54		55 and over		All ages	
	1968	1978	1968	1978	1968	1978	1968	1978	1968	1978	1968	1978
	The North											
	%	%	%	%	%	%	%	%	%	%	%	%
0	29	30	30	29	26	35	24	28	29	23	28	30
1-5	54	51	52	52	57	51	67	56	55	59	56	53
6 or more	17	19	18	19	17	14	9	16	16	18	16	17
Total	100	100	100	100	100	100	100	100	100	100	100	100
Mean	2.7	3.0	2.9	2.9	2.8	2.5	2.4	2.9	2.4	2.9	2.7	2.8
Base	119	148	107	176	101	130	58	98	51	68	436	620
	Wales and the South West											
	%	%	%	%	%	%	%	%	%	%	%	%
0	38	59	34	49	27	53	28	43	(7)	53	32	51
1-5	49	36	48	46	58	43	66	52	(13)	42	54	44
6 or more	13	5	18	5	15	4	6	5	(2)	5	14	5
Total	100	100	100	100	100	100	100	100		100	100	100
Mean	2.3	1.3	3.1	1.3	2.7	1.3	2.5	1.4	*	1.3	2.7	1.3
Base	45	94	62	110	52	95	32	71	(22)	63	213	434
	Midlands and East Anglia											
	%	%	%	%	%	%	%	%	%	%	%	%
0	41	42	33	46	34	44	35	42	36	50	36	45
1-5	48	51	53	47	59	47	51	51	52	39	53	47
6 or more	11	7	14	7	7	9	14	7	12	11	11	8
Total	100	100	100	100	100	100	100	100	100	100	100	100
Mean	2.0	1.6	2.7	1.7	1.9	1.8	2.2	1.6	2.0	2.0	2.2	1.8
Base	88	137	98	147	86	128	51	85	50	92	373	590
	London and the South East											
	%	%	%	%	%	%	%	%	%	%	%	%
0	46	44	44	41	39	43	45	38	45	30	44	40
1-5	48	49	50	53	55	53	44	57	42	64	48	54
6 or more	6	7	6	6	6	4	11	5	13	6	8	6
Total	100	100	100	100	100	100	100	100	100	100	100	100
Mean	1.5	1.7	1.5	1.6	1.9	1.5	2.0	1.5	2.2	1.8	1.8	1.6
Base	119	187	178	208	157	175	116	129	102	143	672	842

* *Percentages and means are not given for bases of less than 30.*

Table 6A.12 Distribution of numbers of decayed teeth among dentate adults in different age groups by dental attendance pattern

No. of decayed teeth	Age											
	16-24		25-34		35-44		45-54		55 and over		All ages	
	1968	1978	1968	1978	1968	1978	1968	1978	1968	1978	1968	1978
	People who go to the dentist for regular check-ups											
	%	%	%	%	%	%	%	%	%	%	%	%
0	51	51	55	52	44	52	49	49	52	48	50	51
1-5	45	43	43	45	52	46	49	49	45	49	47	46
6 or more	4	6	2	3	4	2	2	2	3	3	3	3
Total	100	100	100	100	100	100	100	100	100	100	100	100
Mean	1.1	1.3	1.0	1.1	1.3	1.0	1.2	1.1	1.2	1.1	1.1	1.1
Base	169	263	197	320	164	264	90	171	60	130	680	1148
	People who only go to the dentist when they have trouble with their teeth											
	%	%	%	%	%	%	%	%	%	%	%	%
0	20	30	16	22	20	28	30	29	30	32	23	28
1-5	58	52	62	57	64	56	53	56	52	54	58	55
6 or more	22	18	22	21	16	16	17	15	18	14	19	17
Total	100	100	100	100	100	100	100	100	100	100	100	100
Mean	3.4	2.9	3.7	3.3	3.2	2.9	2.9	2.7	2.8	2.7	3.2	2.9
Base	143	197	191	218	195	197	144	173	144	197	817	983

7 The condition of the individual teeth

In 1968 we looked at the distribution of decay and its treatment around the mouth for all adults who still had some natural teeth and for the two age groups, adults aged 16-34 and adults aged 35 or over. The results were presented in the form of diagrams which showed the proportions of each tooth type that were missing, sound, actively decayed or filled (otherwise sound). The corresponding figures for 1978 are found at the end of this chapter. As in 1968, the figures are made up of the upper and lower jaw with the latter being inverted to represent the mouth. The data from which these figures were constructed can also be found at the end of this chapter.

The figures for 1978 have been produced with the same dimensions as those in the 1968 report so that readers can make a direct comparison if they wish to.

Figure 7.1 shows the distribution of decay and treatment for each tooth type among adults of all ages with some natural teeth. Comparison with the equivalent diagram for 1968 shows that the proportion of teeth present has increased for nearly all tooth types. For each of the front teeth in the upper jaw this proportion has increased by the same amount which reflects the fact that a smaller proportion of people with some natural teeth in 1978 had been found to have a full upper jaw denture. However, the proportion of molars present (except for the wisdom teeth) showed a larger increase between 1968 and 1978 than the proportion of front teeth present, suggesting the influence of other factors, in addition to the decrease in full upper denture wearing. In fact, if we look at the condition of the molars which were present in 1968 and 1978, we can see this increase was largely due to an increase in the proportion which were filled (otherwise sound) suggesting that in 1978, molars, which previously might have been extracted, were being restoratively treated.

The proportion of wisdom teeth present has decreased in both jaws and this decrease was associated with a decrease in the proportion of these teeth which were actively decayed, suggesting that for the wisdom teeth, in contrast to the other molars, a higher proportion were being extracted rather than restoratively treated.

The condition of the front teeth of the lower jaw showed little change in the ten-year period but, as in the upper jaw, there had been an increase in the proportion of molars present which again reflected a rise in the proportion of molars which were filled (otherwise sound).

In the previous chapter we saw that there had been no overall decrease in the proportion of teeth which were actively decayed and from the diagrams we see that this was true for each type of tooth and in both jaws, except for the wisdom teeth where, as noted above, the proportion that were actively decayed had decreased slightly.

If the figures are compared in terms of the proportion of each tooth type recorded as sound and untreated, it will be seen that there is virtually no difference between the two surveys. This emphasises the above results which suggest that for the most part the changes indicated an increase in restorative treatment at the expense of extractive treatment.

Figure 7.2 presents similar data but for dentate adults aged 16-34 rather than people of all ages. Among this group of younger adults, there was some indication that a higher proportion of various tooth types were sound and untreated. This was particularly so among molars and premolars in the upper jaw. It is not possible from the survey results to ascertain whether this increase was the result of a reduction in need for treatment or a reduction in the provision of treatment at stages earlier in the decay process than could be detected by the survey dental examination, resulting in an apparent decrease in the incidence of disease. There was, however, an increase in the proportion of teeth present, which was most noticeable among the 'fives', 'sixes' and 'sevens' in both jaws, where the amount of restorative treatment had increased.

In Figure 7.3, the results are shown for older dentate adults, that is those aged 35 and over. Dental findings for this group need to be interpreted fairly carefully because the group is subject to a wide range of dental influences. It is subject to increasing loss among the older people to edentulousness, and, of course, those who still retain some natural teeth are likely to have partial dentures — some of which will be extensive partial dentures. The figure clearly reflects the situation in the large proportion of teeth which were missing, especially of posterior teeth. The upper jaw is also clearly influenced by the fact that some people in this age group have a full upper denture. In fact, in 1968 18% of this age group had a full upper denture and in 1978 the figure was 14%. The 4% reduction in upper jaw full clearance would appear to account for only about half the difference in missing teeth. It would seem therefore, that there has been an increase in the retention of individual upper teeth. In nearly all the tooth positions in both jaws there was an increase in the proportion of teeth that were filled (otherwise sound). As was said earlier, it is not necessarily the case that these fillings were carried out during the last ten years, but that more people now in this age group have a history of restorative treatment.

The general analysis of the condition of the teeth in Chapter 6 clearly revealed variations for people of different dental attendance patterns and from different regions. In the 1968 report, the condition of the individual tooth types were given for the two main attendance patterns, contrasting the North and London and the South East. The corresponding results for 1978 are shown in Figures 7.4 to 7.11.

Figure 7.4 shows the decay and treatment experience of adults aged 16-34 with some natural teeth, from London and the South East who attend for a regular check-up. Comparing the two surveys we see that in 1978 there were higher proportions of sound and untreated teeth for nearly all tooth types. There was also a decrease in the proportion of filled teeth among premolars and wisdom teeth.

Figure 7.5 shows the finding for young dentate adults in 1978 from London and the South East who only go to the dentist when they have trouble with their teeth. As in 1968, this attendance pattern group had fewer fillings and a higher level of decay than was the case among regular dental attenders. However, compared with the group of the same age and attendance pattern ten years earlier, the 1978 situation was a considerable improvement. The proportion of missing teeth in the upper jaw and among the posterior teeth of the lower jaw was much lower than had been the case in 1968. The proportion of filled teeth was greater and the proportion of sound, untreated teeth had risen.

Figure 7.6 shows the 1978 results for young dentate adults from the North who are regular attenders. For this group there was little change between 1968 and 1978 except for an increase in the proportion of 'sevens' present in both jaws. The increased proportion of 'sevens' present was a feature evident among several of the groups examined. This is perhaps to be expected because, since the 'sixes' have in the past tended to be lost early in life, any

change in treatment patterns towards restoration and retention of molars will be noticeable more quickly among adults in terms of the plight of the 'sevens'.

Figure 7.7 shows the remaining group of young dentate adults, those from the North who only go to the dentist when they are having trouble with their teeth. In 1968 we saw that this group had a low level of fillings and a high level of active decay. In 1978 the level of active decay was still very high but there was a higher proportion of teeth which were filled (otherwise sound). This was most noticeable among the 'sixes' and 'sevens' in both jaws. There was some reduction in the proportion of missing teeth but this was nowhere near the improvement suggested by the results for people with a similar attendance pattern in London and the South East.

Figures 7.8 to 7.11 follow the same pattern as those already described but present the results for the older dentate adults. The regular attenders in London and the South East were, in 1978, retaining more teeth and had more filled teeth especially in the upper jaw. Those who attend only when having trouble with their teeth aged 35 and over in London and the South East were retaining more teeth in all parts of the upper jaw and in the posterior parts of the lower jaw. There was more evidence of restorative work and even some reduction in active decay particularly in the upper jaw. However, the dental prognosis for this group was still grossly inferior to that of the regular attenders.

In the North older dentate regular attenders (Figure 7.10) had fewer missing teeth and less active decay in 1978 than had been the case in 1968. Among older dentate adults who are irregular dental attenders in the North, there were fewer missing teeth in the upper jaw and more filled teeth. In the lower jaw there was an increase in the proportion of lower missing incisors as compared with 1968.

The distribution of tooth conditions around the mouth.

Figure 7.1   *Adults of all ages, with some natural teeth.*

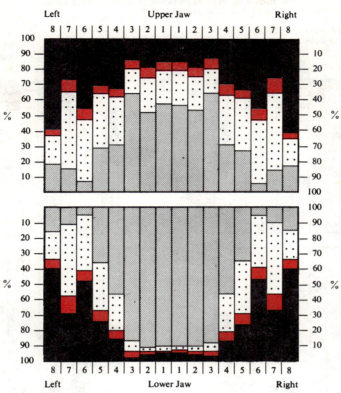

Figure 7. 2 Adults aged 16-34, with some natural teeth.

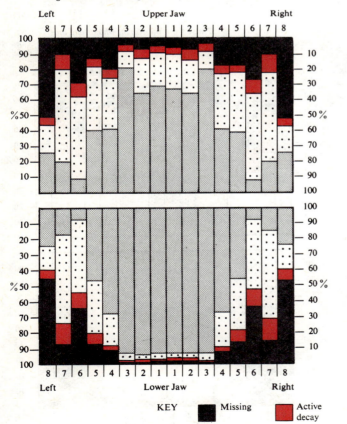

Figure 7. 3 Adults aged 35 or more, with some natural teeth.

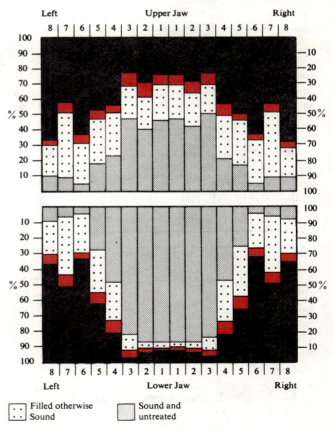

KEY   ■ Missing   ■ Active decay   ⋯ Filled otherwise / Sound   ▦ Sound and untreated

The distribution of tooth conditions around the mouth, for adults
aged 16-34, with some natural teeth.

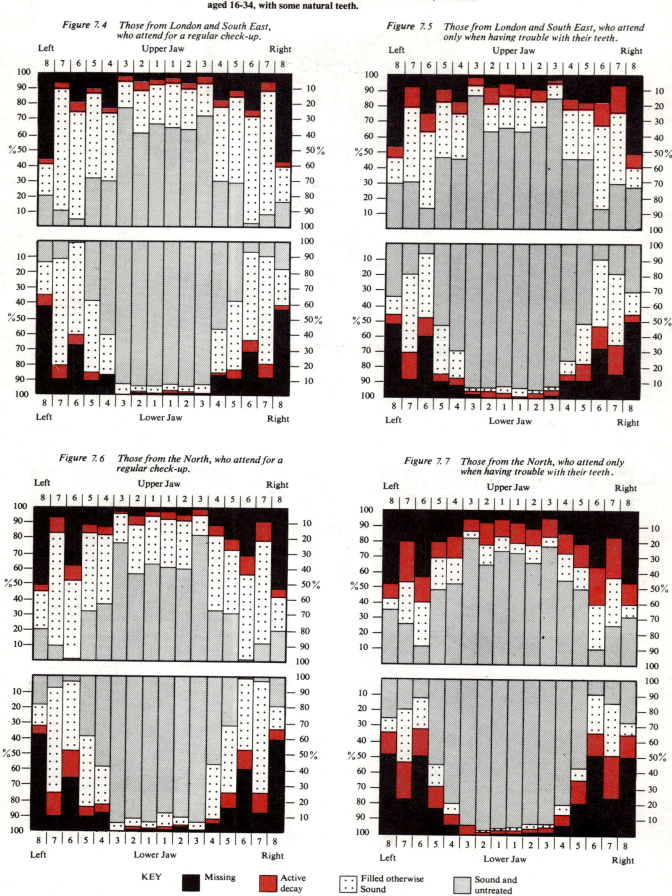

Figure 7.4   Those from London and South East, who attend for a regular check-up.

Figure 7.5   Those from London and South East, who attend only when having trouble with their teeth.

Figure 7.6   Those from the North, who attend for a regular check-up.

Figure 7.7   Those from the North, who attend only when having trouble with their teeth.

KEY   Missing   Active decay   Filled otherwise   Sound   Sound and untreated

The distribution of tooth conditions around the mouth, for adults
aged 35 or more, with some natural teeth.

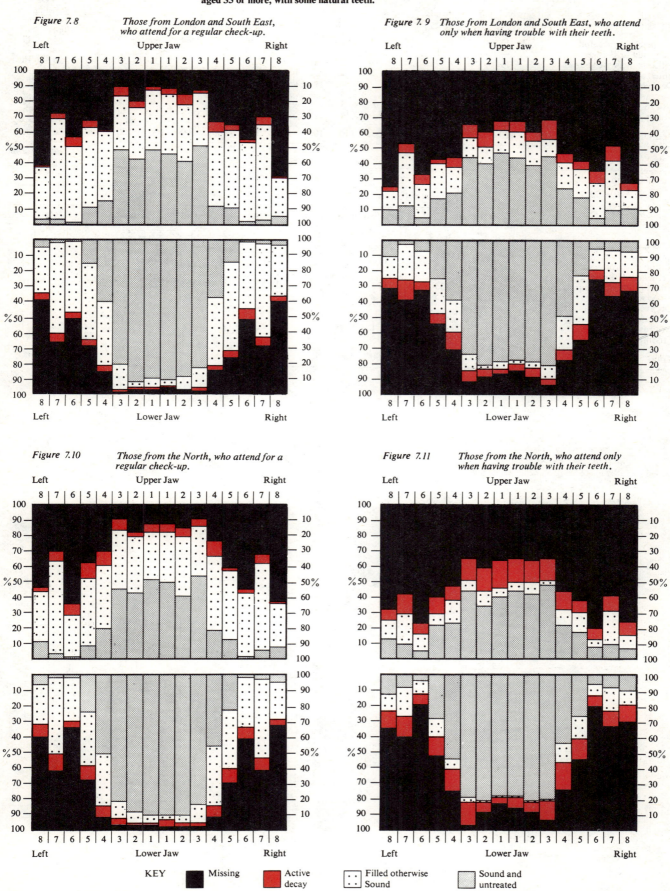

Figure 7.8   Those from London and South East,
who attend for a regular check-up.

Figure 7.9   Those from London and South East, who attend
only when having trouble with their teeth.

Figure 7.10   Those from the North, who attend for a
regular check-up.

Figure 7.11   Those from the North, who attend only
when having trouble with their teeth.

KEY   ■ Missing   ■ Active decay   ⋯ Filled otherwise / Sound   ☐ Sound and untreated

Table 7A.1 All adults in England and Wales with some natural teeth

Upper Jaw

Tooth conditions	Left: Molars 8	7	6	Premolars 5	4	Canine 3	Incisors 2	1	Right: Incisors 1	2	Canine 3	Premolars 4	5	Molars 6	7	8
	%	%	%	%	%	%	%	%	%	%	%	%	%	%	%	%
Sound and untreated	18	15	7	29	31	64	52	57	56	53	64	31	27	6	14	17
Crowned or Bridged	—	—	1	1	1	1	3	5	5	4	1	1	1	1	—	—
Filled (otherwise sound)	19	50	39	34	30	15	19	17	18	18	15	31	33	40	50	18
Filled and decayed	1	4	4	2	2	2	2	1	2	2	2	3	2	4	4	1
Decayed, not previously treated but restorable	2	3	2	2	2	3	4	4	3	3	4	3	2	2	4	2
Not restorable	1	1	1	1	1	1	1	1	1	1	1	1	1	1	2	1
Missing	59	27	46	31	33	14	19	15	15	19	13	30	34	46	26	61
Total	100	100	100	100	100	100	100	100	100	100	100	100	100	100	100	100

Base = 2480

Lower Jaw

Tooth conditions	Left: Molars 8	7	6	Premolars 5	4	Canine 3	Incisors 2	1	Right: Incisors 1	2	Canine 3	Premolars 4	5	Molars 6	7	8
	%	%	%	%	%	%	%	%	%	%	%	%	%	%	%	%
Sound and untreated	16	11	5	36	57	87	91	90	90	90	88	57	35	5	10	15
Crowned or Bridged	—	1	1	1	—	—	—	1	—	1	—	1	1	1	1	—
Filled (otherwise sound)	18	46	35	30	23	7	3	3	3	3	6	24	33	33	46	19
Filled and decayed	2	6	5	3	2	1	—	—	—	—	—	2	3	5	4	2
Decayed, not previously treated but restorable	3	4	1	3	3	2	2	1	2	2	2	3	3	1	4	3
Not restorable	1	1	1	1	1	1	—	—	—	—	1	1	1	2	2	1
Missing	60	31	52	26	14	2	4	5	5	4	3	13	24	53	33	60
Total	100	100	100	100	100	100	100	100	100	100	100	100	100	100	100	100

Base = 2480

Table 7A.2 Adults aged 16-34 with some natural teeth

Tooth conditions	Upper Jaw															
	Left								Right							
	Molars			Premolars		Canine	Incisors				Canine	Premolars		Molars		
	8	7	6	5	4	3	2	1	1	2	3	4	5	6	7	8
	%	%	%	%	%	%	%	%	%	%	%	%	%	%	%	%
Sound and untreated	26	20	9	40	41	81	64	69	67	64	80	41	39	8	20	26
Crowned or Bridged	—	1	1	1	—	1	3	5	5	3	1	1	1	1	—	—
Filled (otherwise sound)	18	59	52	41	33	10	20	17	18	19	11	35	38	55	58	17
Filled and decayed	1	4	5	2	2	1	3	1	2	2	1	2	2	5	4	1
Decayed, not previously treated but restorable	3	5	3	2	3	2	3	3	2	4	3	3	2	3	6	3
Not restorable	1	1	1	1	1	1	—	—	—	1	1	1	1	1	2	1
Missing	51	10	29	13	20	4	7	5	6	7	3	17	17	27	10	52
Total	100	100	100	100	100	100	100	100	100	100	100	100	100	100	100	100

Base = 1205

Tooth conditions	Lower Jaw															
	Left								Right							
	Molars			Premolars		Canine	Incisors				Canine	Premolars		Molars		
	8	7	6	5	4	3	2	1	1	2	3	4	5	6	7	8
	%	%	%	%	%	%	%	%	%	%	%	%	%	%	%	%
Sound and untreated	24	17	7	46	68	93	94	93	93	93	93	67	45	7	14	23
Crowned or Bridged	—	1	1	—	—	—	—	—	—	—	—	—	—	—	—	—
Filled (otherwise sound)	15	56	46	34	20	5	3	4	3	3	5	22	33	45	57	16
Filled and decayed	1	7	7	3	1	—	—	—	—	1	—	1	3	7	6	2
Decayed, not previously treated but restorable	4	5	2	3	2	1	2	1	2	1	1	2	4	2	6	4
Not restorable	1	1	1	1	—	—	—	—	—	—	—	—	1	2	2	1
Missing	55	13	36	13	9	1	1	2	2	2	1	8	14	37	15	54
Total	100	100	100	100	100	100	100	100	100	100	100	100	100	100	100	100

Base = 1205

Table 7A.3 Adults aged 35 or more with some natural teeth

Tooth conditions	Upper Jaw															
	Left								Right							
	Molars			Premolars		Canine	Incisors				Canine	Premolars		Molars		
	8	7	6	5	4	3	2	1	1	2	3	4	5	6	7	8
	%	%	%	%	%	%	%	%	%	%	%	%	%	%	%	%
Sound and untreated	10	9	5	18	23	47	40	46	47	42	50	21	17	5	9	9
Crowned or Bridged	—	—	—	1	1	1	3	5	5	5	1	—	1	1	1	—
Filled (otherwise sound)	20	42	26	28	27	20	18	18	17	17	18	28	28	27	41	19
Filled and decayed	1	4	4	2	2	3	2	2	2	2	2	3	2	2	3	1
Decayed, not previously treated but restorable	1	2	1	2	2	5	5	4	4	3	5	3	1	1	2	2
Not restorable	1	1	1	2	1	1	2	1	1	2	1	2	1	1	1	1
Missing	67	42	63	47	44	23	30	24	24	29	23	43	50	63	43	68
Total	100	100	100	100	100	100	100	100	100	100	100	100	100	100	100	100

Base = 1274

Tooth conditions	Lower Jaw															
	Left								Right							
	Molars			Premolars		Canine	Incisors				Canine	Premolars		Molars		
	8	7	6	5	4	3	2	1	1	2	3	4	5	6	7	8
	%	%	%	%	%	%	%	%	%	%	%	%	%	%	%	%
Sound and untreated	9	6	4	27	48	82	87	87	87	87	84	47	25	4	6	8
Crowned or Bridged	—	1	1	1	—	1	1	1	1	—	—	1	1	—	1	—
Filled (otherwise sound)	21	36	24	27	25	9	3	3	2	4	8	27	32	21	35	22
Filled and decayed	3	5	2	3	3	1	—	—	—	—	—	3	3	3	4	2
Decayed, not previously treated but restorable	2	2	1	3	3	3	2	1	2	2	3	4	3	1	2	2
Not restorable	1	1	1	1	2	1	1	—	—	1	1	1	2	2	1	1
Missing	64	49	67	38	19	3	6	8	8	6	4	18	34	68	51	65
Total	100	100	100	100	100	100	100	100	100	100	100	100	100	100	100	100

Base = 1274

Table 7A.4 Those from London & the South East who attend for a regular check-up, adults aged 16-34 with some natural teeth

Upper Jaw

Tooth conditions	Molars			Premolars		Canine	Incisors				Canine	Premolars		Molars		
	8	7	6	5	4	3	2	1	1	2	3	4	5	6	7	8
	%	%	%	%	%	%	%	%	%	%	%	%	%	%	%	%
Sound and untreated	20	11	5	32	30	78	61	67	65	64	73	30	29	3	9	17
Crowned or Bridged	—	1	1	2	1	2	5	6	7	6	—	2	3	2	—	—
Filled (otherwise sound)	21	78	70	53	44	15	23	20	22	20	21	47	53	68	80	23
Filled and decayed	1	3	4	2	2	2	4	2	2	2	2	1	2	3	4	—
Decayed, not previously treated but restorable	2	1	1	1	1	—	2	1	1	2	2	2	2	1	2	3
Not restorable	—	—	—	—	—	1	—	—	—	—	—	1	—	—	—	—
Missing	56	6	19	10	22	2	5	4	3	6	2	17	11	23	5	57
Total	100	100	100	100	100	100	100	100	100	100	100	100	100	100	100	100

Base = 178

Lower Jaw

Tooth conditions	Molars			Premolars		Canine	Incisors				Canine	Premolars		Molars		
	8	7	6	5	4	3	2	1	1	2	3	4	5	6	7	8
	%	%	%	%	%	%	%	%	%	%	%	%	%	%	%	%
Sound and untreated	14	12	1	39	61	93	94	94	93	94	93	57	38	6	9	17
Crowned or Bridged	—	1	3	—	—	—	1	2	11	1	1	—	1	1	1	—
Filled (otherwise sound)	21	68	57	47	26	7	3	3	3	3	5	28	44	57	69	23
Filled and decayed	3	7	6	4	—	—	—	—	1	—	—	—	4	7	6	2
Decayed, not previously treated but restorable	4	2	1	1	—	—	1	—	1	1	—	1	2	—	2	1
Not restorable	—	—	—	—	—	—	—	—	—	—	—	1	—	—	1	—
Missing	58	10	32	9	13	—	1	1	1	1	1	13	11	29	12	57
Total	100	100	100	100	100	100	100	100	100	100	100	100	100	100	100	100

Base = 178

Table 7A.5 Those from London & the South East who attend only when having trouble, adults aged 16-34 with some natural teeth

Upper Jaw

Tooth conditions	Molars			Premolars		Canine	Incisors				Canine	Premolars		Molars		
	8	7	6	5	4	3	2	1	1	2	3	4	5	6	7	8
	%	%	%	%	%	%	%	%	%	%	%	%	%	%	%	%
Sound and untreated	30	31	14	47	46	87	64	66	64	67	85	46	46	14	30	28
Crowned or Bridged	—	2	1	—	—	2	3	5	5	2	2	1	—	—	—	—
Filled (otherwise sound)	17	47	49	36	30	5	15	16	17	15	8	32	33	54	47	13
Filled and decayed	1	3	4	4	2	—	5	2	2	3	—	3	2	8	5	2
Decayed, not previously treated but restorable	4	8	5	2	3	4	5	6	3	4	1	1	1	3	9	5
Not restorable	2	2	3	2	2	1	1	—	1	—	1	2	1	4	3	2
Missing	46	7	24	9	17	1	7	5	8	9	3	15	17	17	6	50
Total	100	100	100	100	100	100	100	100	100	100	100	100	100	100	100	100

Base = 131

Lower Jaw

Tooth conditions	Molars			Premolars		Canine	Incisors				Canine	Premolars		Molars		
	8	7	6	5	4	3	2	1	1	2	3	4	5	6	7	8
	%	%	%	%	%	%	%	%	%	%	%	%	%	%	%	%
Sound and untreated	35	20	7	54	70	94	94	93	94	95	93	76	52	10	19	31
Crowned or Bridged	—	1	1	—	—	—	1	1	1	—	2	—	1	—	1	—
Filled (otherwise sound)	12	50	40	31	18	2	1	3	4	2	2	8	26	43	47	14
Filled and decayed	1	9	9	2	1	—	1	1	—	2	—	1	4	7	8	2
Decayed, not previously treated but restorable	5	7	2	2	3	2	3	2	1	1	2	2	3	3	8	2
Not restorable	—	2	2	1	—	—	—	—	—	—	1	1	4	4	3	1
Missing	47	11	39	10	8	2	—	—	—	—	2	11	11	32	15	50
Total	100	100	100	100	100	100	100	100	100	100	100	100	100	100	100	100

Base = 131

Table 7A.6 Those from the North who attend for a regular check-up, adults aged 16-34 with some natural teeth

Tooth conditions	Upper Jaw															
	Left								Right							
	Molars			Premolars		Canine	Incisors				Canine	Premolars		Molars		
	8	7	6	5	4	3	2	1	1	2	3	4	5	6	7	8
	%	%	%	%	%	%	%	%	%	%	%	%	%	%	%	%
Sound and untreated	20	10	1	32	37	77	56	63	61	60	82	33	31	1	12	20
Crowned or Bridged	—	—	1	1	1	1	4	7	9	4	—	—	1	—	—	—
Filled (otherwise sound)	25	73	50	50	44	18	28	24	22	27	13	49	41	55	67	22
Filled and decayed	1	7	9	3	3	—	4	2	4	2	1	3	6	11	5	2
Decayed, not previously treated but restorable	3	3	1	2	1	1	2	1	1	2	3	3	1	2	5	3
Not restorable	—	—	—	—	1	—	—	—	—	—	—	—	—	—	1	—
Missing	51	7	38	12	13	3	6	3	3	5	1	12	20	31	10	53
Total	100	100	100	100	100	100	100	100	100	100	100	100	100	100	100	100

Base = 144

Tooth conditions	Lower Jaw															
	Left								Right							
	Molars			Premolars		Canine	Incisors				Canine	Premolars		Molars		
	8	7	6	5	4	3	2	1	1	2	3	4	5	6	7	8
	%	%	%	%	%	%	%	%	%	%	%	%	%	%	%	%
Sound and untreated	19	8	4	39	59	95	92	94	89	91	94	57	32	1	3	19
Crowned or Bridged	—	1	1	—	—	—	—	—	1	1	1	—	—	—	—	—
Filled (otherwise sound)	14	67	43	46	24	5	5	4	8	4	4	35	43	46	72	15
Filled and decayed	2	12	18	4	1	—	1	—	1	—	—	1	6	11	10	3
Decayed, not previously treated but restorable	3	2	—	1	5	—	1	1	1	1	—	2	4	1	3	3
Not restorable	—	1	—	1	—	—	—	—	—	—	—	—	—	1	—	—
Missing	62	9	34	9	11	—	1	1	1	3	1	5	15	40	12	60
Total	100	100	100	100	100	100	100	100	100	100	100	100	100	100	100	100

Base = 144

Table 7A.7 Those from the North who attend only when having trouble, adults aged 16-34 with some natural teeth

Tooth conditions	Upper Jaw															
	Left								Right							
	Molars			Premolars		Canine	Incisors				Canine	Premolars		Molars		
	8	7	6	5	4	3	2	1	1	2	3	4	5	6	7	8
	%	%	%	%	%	%	%	%	%	%	%	%	%	%	%	%
Sound and untreated	35	26	12	48	52	82	65	74	73	66	77	54	49	11	25	31
Crowned or Bridged	—	—	—	—	—	2	5	2	3	—	—	—	—	—	—	—
Filled (otherwise sound)	7	27	28	21	17	4	11	4	4	9	6	19	15	28	31	8
Filled and decayed	2	8	7	2	3	1	4	3	2	—	2	3	4	11	5	1
Decayed, not previously treated but restorable	6	14	5	7	6	6	8	6	9	7	8	7	8	11	15	8
Not restorable	2	5	4	2	5	1	2	2	2	3	2	2	3	3	7	5
Missing	48	20	44	20	17	6	8	6	8	12	5	15	21	36	17	47
Total	100	100	100	100	100	100	100	100	100	100	100	100	100	100	100	100

Base = 132

Tooth conditions	Lower Jaw															
	Left								Right							
	Molars			Premolars		Canine	Incisors				Canine	Premolars		Molars		
	8	7	6	5	4	3	2	1	1	2	3	4	5	6	7	8
	%	%	%	%	%	%	%	%	%	%	%	%	%	%	%	%
Sound and untreated	25	19	12	55	80	94	97	96	95	93	93	80	57	9	15	28
Crowned or Bridged	—	—	—	—	—	—	—	—	—	—	—	—	—	—	—	—
Filled (otherwise sound)	9	35	20	14	7	—	1	1	2	3	2	7	8	25	33	7
Filled and decayed	2	4	5	2	1	—	—	1	—	1	2	1	3	6	6	—
Decayed, not previously treated but restorable	8	12	8	10	5	4	1	1	2	1	1	5	10	6	17	11
Not restorable	4	7	4	2	1	—	1	—	—	—	—	1	1	2	5	3
Missing	52	23	51	17	6	2	—	1	1	2	2	6	21	52	24	51
Total	100	100	100	100	100	100	100	100	100	100	100	100	100	100	100	100

Base = 132

Table 7A.8 Those from London & the South East who attend for a regular check-up, adults aged 35 or more with some natural teeth

Tooth conditions	Upper Jaw															
	Left								Right							
	Molars			Premolars		Canine	Incisors				Canine	Premolars		Molars		
	8	7	6	5	4	3	2	1	1	2	3	4	5	6	7	8
	%	%	%	%	%	%	%	%	%	%	%	%	%	%	%	%
Sound and untreated	3	3	1	11	15	48	42	48	46	41	51	12	11	2	3	6
Crowned or Bridged	—	1	1	2	2	2	6	10	10	9	3	2	2	2	—	—
Filled (otherwise sound)	34	64	48	50	43	33	28	29	28	28	31	46	48	49	62	25
Filled and decayed	1	4	6	2	1	4	2	2	4	4	2	5	4	2	5	—
Decayed, not previously treated but restorable	—	—	—	1	—	2	2	—	—	2	—	2	—	—	—	1
Not restorable	—	—	—	1	—	—	—	—	—	—	—	—	—	—	—	—
Missing	62	28	44	33	39	11	20	11	12	16	13	33	35	45	30	68
Total	100	100	100	100	100	100	100	100	100	100	100	100	100	100	100	100

Base = 216

Tooth conditions	Lower Jaw															
	Left								Right							
	Molars			Premolars		Canine	Incisors				Canine	Premolars		Molars		
	8	7	6	5	4	3	2	1	1	2	3	4	5	6	7	8
	%	%	%	%	%	%	%	%	%	%	%	%	%	%	%	%
Sound and untreated	5	2	1	16	40	81	92	90	91	89	84	38	15	1	3	4
Crowned or Bridged	1	1	2	3	2	2	1	2	1	2	1	1	2	3	1	—
Filled (otherwise sound)	29	58	44	46	40	14	3	4	3	6	11	43	55	41	60	33
Filled and decayed	4	5	4	3	2	1	—	—	—	—	1	3	5	6	5	2
Decayed, not previously treated but restorable	—	1	—	1	2	1	1	1	1	—	1	—	—	1	—	1
Not restorable	—	—	—	—	—	—	—	—	—	—	—	—	—	—	—	—
Missing	61	33	49	31	14	1	3	3	4	3	2	15	23	48	31	60
Total	100	100	100	100	100	100	100	100	100	100	100	100	100	100	100	100

Base = 216

Table 7A.9 Those from London & the South East who attend only when having trouble, adults aged 35 or more with some natural teeth

Tooth conditions	Upper Jaw															
	Left								Right							
	Molars			Premolars		Canine	Incisors				Canine	Premolars		Molars		
	8	7	6	5	4	3	2	1	1	2	3	4	5	6	7	8
	%	%	%	%	%	%	%	%	%	%	%	%	%	%	%	%
Sound and untreated	10	13	5	17	21	44	40	47	44	39	45	24	18	5	10	11
Crowned or Bridged	—	1	1	1	1	1	3	3	3	3	2	1	2	1	1	—
Filled (otherwise sound)	12	33	20	22	16	12	8	12	14	13	9	16	17	22	32	12
Filled and decayed	1	5	5	1	2	4	4	2	2	2	4	2	1	3	5	1
Decayed, not previously treated but restorable	1	1	1	—	2	4	4	4	4	2	7	2	3	3	3	3
Not restorable	1	—	1	2	2	1	2	—	1	2	2	2	1	2	1	1
Missing	75	47	67	57	56	34	39	32	32	39	31	53	58	64	48	72
Total	100	100	100	100	100	100	100	100	100	100	100	100	100	100	100	100

Base = 171

Tooth conditions	Lower Jaw															
	Left								Right							
	Molars			Premolars		Canine	Incisors				Canine	Premolars		Molars		
	8	7	6	5	4	3	2	1	1	2	3	4	5	6	7	8
	%	%	%	%	%	%	%	%	%	%	%	%	%	%	%	%
Sound and untreated	11	3	7	26	39	74	81	79	78	79	81	49	23	5	6	7
Crowned or Bridged	—	1	1	—	—	1	1	1	—	1	1	1	2	1	2	1
Filled (otherwise sound)	15	23	20	22	21	10	2	4	2	3	8	21	30	13	20	16
Filled and decayed	4	8	3	4	4	1	1	—	1	1	1	5	3	3	2	4
Decayed, not previously treated but restorable	1	2	1	2	3	4	3	3	3	3	2	1	4	1	2	4
Not restorable	1	2	1	1	4	2	1	—	1	2	1	1	3	3	4	1
Missing	68	61	67	45	29	8	11	13	15	11	6	22	35	74	64	67
Total	100	100	100	100	100	100	100	100	100	100	100	100	100	100	100	100

Base 171

Table 7A.10 Those from the North who attend for a regular check-up, adults aged 35 or more with some natural teeth

Tooth conditions	Upper Jaw															
	Left								Right							
	Molars			Premolars		Canine	Incisors				Canine	Premolars		Molars		
	8	7	6	5	4	3	2	1	1	2	3	4	5	6	7	8
	%	%	%	%	%	%	%	%	%	%	%	%	%	%	%	%
Sound and untreated	11	3	1	8	19	45	42	51	49	40	53	18	12	1	5	7
Crowned or Bridged	—	—	—	1	2	4	6	4	5	8	1	—	1	—	2	—
Filled (otherwise sound)	32	60	27	43	39	34	31	27	28	31	31	48	43	41	54	28
Filled and decayed	3	5	4	6	9	4	2	4	3	3	4	10	1	2	4	1
Decayed, not previously treated but restorable	—	—	3	2	—	3	1	1	2	2	1	—	—	1	1	—
Not restorable	—	1	—	2	—	—	—	—	—	—	—	—	1	—	1	—
Missing	54	31	65	38	31	10	18	13	13	16	10	24	42	55	33	64
Total	100	100	100	100	100	100	100	100	100	100	100	100	100	100	100	100

Base = 114

Tooth conditions	Lower Jaw															
	Left								Right							
	Molars			Premolars		Canine	Incisors				Canine	Premolars		Molars		
	8	7	6	5	4	3	2	1	1	2	3	4	5	6	7	8
	%	%	%	%	%	%	%	%	%	%	%	%	%	%	%	%
Sound and untreated	6	2	2	24	51	82	89	91	91	91	84	46	23	2	3	5
Crowned or Bridged	—	—	1	2	—	—	—	—	—	—	—	—	1	1	—	—
Filled (otherwise sound)	26	49	27	33	34	11	7	5	3	5	12	39	37	31	51	24
Filled and decayed	6	10	3	6	4	1	1	—	3	1	—	2	7	7	7	4
Decayed, not previously treated but restorable	2	1	1	3	3	3	—	1	1	1	2	5	2	—	1	—
Not restorable	—	—	—	—	—	—	—	—	—	—	—	—	—	1	—	—
Missing	60	38	66	32	8	3	3	3	2	2	2	8	30	58	38	67
Total	100	100	100	100	100	100	100	100	100	100	100	100	100	100	100	100

Base = 114

Table 7A.11 Those from the North who attend only when having trouble, adults aged 35 or more with some natural teeth

Tooth conditions	Upper Jaw															
	Left								Right							
	Molars			Premolars		Canine	Incisors				Canine	Premolars		Molars		
	8	7	6	5	4	3	2	1	1	2	3	4	5	6	7	8
	%	%	%	%	%	%	%	%	%	%	%	%	%	%	%	%
Sound and untreated	13	10	5	22	23	44	34	40	44	42	48	22	17	8	10	7
Crowned or Bridged	—	—	—	—	—	—	—	1	1	1	—	—	—	—	—	—
Filled (otherwise sound)	12	19	11	7	15	7	10	5	5	7	3	10	13	5	21	8
Filled and decayed	1	3	3	3	4	2	1	3	1	3	1	3	1	1	2	2
Decayed, not previously treated but restorable	5	7	1	7	5	11	11	12	11	7	11	6	4	3	5	4
Not restorable	1	3	3	1	—	1	3	3	3	4	2	3	3	3	3	3
Missing	68	58	77	60	53	35	41	36	35	36	35	56	62	80	59	76
Total	100	100	100	100	100	100	100	100	100	100	100	100	100	100	100	100

Base = 150

Tooth conditions	Lower Jaw															
	Left								Right							
	Molars			Premolars		Canine	Incisors				Canine	Premolars		Molars		
	8	7	6	5	4	3	2	1	1	2	3	4	5	6	7	8
	%	%	%	%	%	%	%	%	%	%	%	%	%	%	%	%
Sound and untreated	12	8	4	28	54	79	81	78	78	81	80	44	27	6	8	10
Crowned or Bridged	—	—	—	—	—	—	—	—	—	—	—	—	—	—	—	—
Filled (otherwise sound)	11	19	8	12	7	3	1	1	1	1	1	12	14	7	15	9
Filled and decayed	1	6	3	2	2	1	—	—	—	1	1	—	1	3	3	4
Decayed, not previously treated but restorable	8	5	3	8	10	12	5	3	6	4	10	15	7	1	7	5
Not restorable	2	2	1	2	2	2	2	1	1	2	2	3	5	3	—	2
Missing	66	60	81	48	25	3	11	17	14	11	6	26	46	80	67	70
Total	100	100	100	100	100	100	100	100	100	100	100	100	100	100	100	100

Base = 150

8 Changes in dental attitudes

8.1 Introduction

The preceding chapters have shown that the dental health of adults in England and Wales is changing and, indeed, improving. On the whole the changes we have seen have reflected changes in treatment rather than actual levels of disease. (The latter probably requires a rather longer time period than ten years in which to manifest itself). Since dental treatment involves the interaction of a dentist and his patient any change can stem from either the dental profession, the general population or a combination of both. People can influence the type of treatment they receive by how often they attend the dentist, the care they, themselves, take of their mouths and, to some extent, by their expectations and demands. These will in turn be influenced by their general dental attitudes. Once they are in the surgery, however, the treatment they receive will be very much the dentist's decision.

The main evidence of change we have been considering so far has come from the survey dental examination but for investigating changes in attitudes and treatment experience it is clearly appropriate to use the information from the interview.

8.2 Dental attendance pattern and tooth cleaning

As we have said, the two direct influences individuals have on their dental condition are the care they take in such things as teeth cleaning and their dental attendance pattern. We saw in 1968 and again earlier in this report how important dental attendance pattern is with respect to the condition of the natural teeth, so any change in this variable could possibly be one factor which could lead to changes in dental treatment.

The informants were asked if, in general, they went to the dentist for a regular check-up, an occasional check-up or only when they were having trouble with their teeth. This question was identical to that asked in the 1968 survey.

In 1968, one in two people said they only went to the dentist if they had trouble with their teeth. This proportion had decreased to 40% by 1978 with a larger proportion saying they went for regular check-ups and slightly more who said they went for occasional check-ups. These changes varied with age. Although a greater proportion of people aged 35 or more said they went for regular check-ups, the apparent changes in the younger age groups wree not found to be statistically significant. However, the 16 to 24 year olds were the only group who did not show a large reduction in the proportion who said they went to the dentist only when they had trouble with their teeth.

The proportion of people who said they only went to the

Table 8.1 Dental attendance pattern for dentate people in different age groups in 1968 and 1978 in England and Wales

Dental attendance pattern	Age											
	16-24		25-34		35-44		45-54		55 and over		All ages	
	1968	1978	1968	1978	1968	1978	1968	1978	1968	1978	1968	1978
	%	%	%	%	%	%	%	%	%	%	%	%
Regular check-up	46	47	45	50	42	50	35	45	27	36	40	46
Occasional check-up	15	18	12	16	9	12	9	10	8	10	11	14
Only with trouble	39	35	43	34	49	38	56	45	65	54	49	40
Total	100	100	100	100	100	100	100	100	100	100	100	100
Base	*371*	*567*	*445*	*641*	*396*	*528*	*257*	*383*	*225*	*367*	*1694*	*2486*

Table 8.2 Dental attendance pattern for dentate people in different regions in 1968 and 1978

Dental attendance pattern	The North		Wales & the South West		Midlands & East Anglia		London & the South East		England & Wales	
	1968	1978	1968	1978	1968	1978	1968	1978	1968	1978
	%	%	%	%	%	%	%	%	%	%
Regular check-up	37	42	37	49	40	48	45	47	40	46
Occasional check-up	10	13	16	14	8	11	11	17	11	14
Only with trouble	53	45	47	37	52	41	44	36	49	40
Total	100	100	100	100	100	100	100	100	100	100
Base	*436*	*620*	*213*	*434*	*373*	*590*	*672*	*842*	*1694*	*2486*

dentist when having trouble with their teeth had decreased in all regions resulting in the overall regional differences being much the same in 1978 as they had been in 1968. The proportion of regular attenders showed more variability with time and region arising from a large increase in the proportion of regular dental attenders in Wales and the South West and very little change at all in this proportion among people in London and the South East. This latter region was the only one, however, where there had been an increase in the proportion of people who said they went for occasional check-ups. An investigation of the increase in regular attenders in Wales and the South West showed that while for all regions there had in general been an increase among people in equivalent age groups in 1968 and in 1978, in Wales and the South West there also seemed to have been an increase within age cohorts in the proportion of regular attenders.

We asked informants in both surveys how often they cleaned their teeth. It must be borne in mind, of course, that an interview question such as this can take no account of the efficiency of individuals' efforts and so should be used as an indicator of the care people were attempting to take of their teeth rather than any measure of the efficiency with which they were doing it.

The 1978 survey showed that people said they cleaned their teeth more often than was the case in 1968. Nearly two in three dentate adults said they cleaned their teeth twice or more a day in 1978 compared to one in two in 1968. Neither of the surveys had found much variation with age for people aged less than 55 so most of the overall change stemmed from a change within age cohorts over the last ten years. One must assume that any change over

the last ten years or, indeed, prior to that, was probably due not only to the efforts of the dental profession but also to the manufacturers of toothpaste and toothbrushes and their advertising managers. This is also demonstrated by the response to the question on fluoride toothpaste.

Since in 1968 very few toothpastes contained fluoride, while by 1978 nearly all did, this question was designed more to examine the informant's knowledge than to establish the type of toothpaste they used. In the 1978 survey we asked people whether or not the toothpaste they were using contained fluoride with the specific instruction to the interviewers that the informants were not to go and check. Thus 64% of people knew that their toothpaste contained fluoride and although there were still 25% who did not know this must still reflect the influence of advertising campaigns since the introduction of fluoride toothpaste.

Table 8.4 **Whether toothpaste used contains fluoride**

Informant uses toothpaste which:	Adults with some natural teeth	
	1968	1978
	%	%
Contains fluoride	18	64
Does not	55	11
Don't know	27	25
Total	100	100
Base	*1854*	*2912*

8.3 Dental attitudes among the dentate population
We have seen that the care people take of their teeth has improved over the last ten years so it seems likely that this may have been concomitant with a change in attitude towards the loss of the natural teeth. We now go on to in-

Table 8.3 **Frequency of tooth cleaning among dentate adults in different age groups in 1968 and 1978**

Frequency of tooth cleaning	Age											
	16-24		25-34		35-44		45-54		55 and over		All ages	
	1968	1978	1968	1978	1968	1978	1968	1978	1968	1978	1968	1978
	%	%	%	%	%	%	%	%	%	%	%	%
Once a day	35	24	37	25	35	25	36	28	36	33	36	27
Twice a day	45	53	46	53	45	52	44	47	36	44	44	50
More than twice a day	8	17	6	14	8	14	6	16	8	11	7	14
Other qualified answers	11	6	10	7	10	8	10	8	13	7	11	7
Never	1	—	1	1	2	1	4	1	7	5	2	2
Total	100	100	100	100	100	100	100	100	100	100	100	100
Base	*391*	*634*	*480*	*729*	*429*	*610*	*282*	*454*	*272*	*481*	*1854**	*2912**

* Table 8.3 onwards includes all people who took part in the interview.

Table 8.5 **Attitude to full dentures among dentate adults in different age groups**

Finds the thought of full dentures:	Age											
	16-24		25-34		35-44		45-54		55 and over		All ages	
	1968	1978	1968	1978	1968	1978	1968	1978	1968	1978	1968	1978
	%	%	%	%	%	%	%	%	%	%	%	%
Very upsetting	31	54	23	53	30	47	27	43	24	38	27	48
A little upsetting	30	26	30	24	32	25	30	27	28	23	30	25
Not at all upsetting	39	20	47	23	38	28	43	30	48	39	43	27
Total	100	100	100	100	100	100	100	100	100	100	100	100
Base	*391*	*634*	*480*	*729*	*429*	*610*	*282*	*454*	*272*	*481*	*1854*	*2912*

vestigate this using the information from two questions: 'Do you find the thought of losing all your own teeth and having full dentures very upsetting, a little upsetting or not at all upsetting?' and 'If you went to the dentist with an aching back/front tooth would you prefer the dentist to take it out or fill it?'

The proportion of people who found the thought of losing all their teeth and having full dentures very upsetting had nearly doubled between the 1968 survey and the 1978 survey and this was matched by a large reduction in the proportion who thought it was not at all upsetting (Table 8.5). This change was apparent for every age group being most marked among the 25 to 34 year olds. Although there wre more people in every age group who found it upsetting it was people in the oldest age group who found the thought of full dentures least upsetting.

In 1968, 68% of people said that if they had an aching front tooth they would prefer it to be filled and 52% said this when asked about a back tooth. In 1978 these proportion had increased to 81% and 65% respectively (Table 8.6). Thus although there was an increase in the preference for conservative treatment, one in every three people still preferred extractions for aching back teeth. Since we saw in 1968 that there was, in fact, a fair degree of correlation between people's preferences and their treatment experiences, we now go on to look at how this proportion varied in a little more detail.

The proportion of people who preferred an extraction for an aching tooth had decreased for every age group (Table 8.7), although it was still higher among people in the older age groups than among the younger adults. Only 8% of people aged 16 to 24 said they would prefer an aching front tooth to be extracted compared to 31% of adults aged 55 or more. There had also been a decrease within age cohorts in the proportion preferring extraction. For example 38% of 16 to 24 year olds in 1968 would have preferred an aching back tooth to be extracted compared with only 28% of 25 to 34 year olds in 1978. The decrease seen overall arose from decreases among both men and women so that there was still a smaller proportion of women than of men who said they would prefer an extraction for an aching tooth.

We have already seen how dental attendance pattern has

Table 8.6 Preference for extraction versus filling in front and back teeth among dentate adults

Would prefer an aching front/back tooth to be:	Front tooth		Back tooth	
	1968	1978	1968	1978
	%	%	%	%
Extracted	29	17	44	33
Filled	68	81	52	65
Other qualified answer	3	2	4	2
Total	100	100	100	100
Base	*1854*	*2912*	*1854*	*2912*

Table 8.7 Preference for extraction among dentate adults in different age groups and by sex

Age/Sex	Proportion of dentate adults who would prefer an aching tooth to be extracted							
	Front tooth				Back tooth			
	1968		1978		1968		1978	
16-24	16%	*391*	8%	*634*	38%	*391*	22%	*634*
25-34	25%	*480*	12%	*729*	41%	*480*	28%	*729*
35-44	30%	*429*	17%	*610*	45%	*429*	34%	*610*
45-54	32%	*282*	21%	*454*	45%	*282*	38%	*454*
55 or more	48%	*272*	31%	*481*	55%	*272*	47%	*481*
Male	33%	*927*	21%	*1445*	48%	*927*	35%	*1445*
Female	24%	*927*	13%	*1467*	40%	*927*	30%	*1467*

Table 8.8 Preference for extraction among dentate adults by region and dental attendance pattern

	Proportion of dentate adults who would prefer an aching tooth to be extracted							
	Front tooth				Back tooth			
	1968		1978		1968		1978	
	Those who attend for a regular check-up							
The North	4%	*170*	5%	*282*	17%	*170*	15%	*282*
Wales & the South West	12%	*84*	4%	*233*	26%	*84*	16%	*233*
Midlands & East Anglia	8%	*155*	8%	*299*	15%	*155*	16%	*299*
London & the South East	9%	*310*	3%	*451*	15%	*310*	9%	*451*
England & Wales	8%	*719*	5%	*1265*	17%	*719*	13%	*1265*
	Those who attend only when having trouble with their teeth							
The North	45%	*254*	35%	*357*	72%	*254*	60%	*357*
Wales & the South West	49%	*122*	32%	*192*	67%	*122*	60%	*192*
Midlands & East Anglia	64%	*220*	39%	*288*	83%	*220*	66%	*288*
London & the South East	40%	*326*	23%	*393*	60%	*326*	43%	*393*
England & Wales	48%	*922*	32%	*1230*	69%	*922*	56%	*1230*

changed over the last ten years and Table 8.8 shows how the attitudes of different types of dental attenders has changed in England and Wales and the different regions. As one would expect, in 1968 we found that people who went to the dentist regularly were far less likely to express a preference for an extraction than those who only went when they had trouble with their teeth. This being so there was far more scope for a change of attitude among this latter group which is what we in fact found. In 1968, 48% of people who only went to the dentist when they had trouble with their teeth said they would prefer an aching front tooth to be extracted. This figure had decreased to 32% in 1978. There was a similar decrease in the proportion who preferred extraction for back teeth although at 56% in 1978 these irregular dental attenders still displayed a somewhat different attitude from the regular dental attenders of whom 13% said they would prefer an extraction. This change of attitude among the irregular dental attenders is particularly interesting given that the largest increase in the evidence of conservative treatment was found among people in this dental attendance group.

Among the regular dental attenders there had been no change in the proportion of people in the North and the Midlands and East Anglia who preferred extractions. In the other two regions, however, this proportion had decreased for both front and back teeth. Thus in 1978, only 3% of regular dental attenders in London and the South East said they would prefer an aching front tooth to be extracted. The proportion of people who preferred extractions among those who only went to the dentist when they had trouble with their teeth had decreased in every region. This decrease was most marked in the Midlands and East Anglia where 64% of irregular dental attenders had said in 1968 that they would prefer an aching front tooth extracted, compared to 39% in 1978. Even with this large decrease, however, people in the Midlands and East Anglia who only went to the dentist when they had trouble with their teeth still showed the highest preference for extractions.

8.4 The most recent course of treatment

We have seen that, in general, people now seem to be more concerned with the preservation of their teeth. The analysis of the dental examination data showed that in 1978 there were fewer missing teeth and more filled teeth

than in 1968. Thus one might expect that the pattern of treatment within individual courses of treatment may also have changed which can in fact be seen in Table 8.9. It is, of course, not possible to tell from survey data to what extent this change is due to a change in people's attitudes, a change in the course of treatment decided upon by the dentist, or a change in the actual levels of disease.

In 1968, the types of treatment received were summarised as shown in Table 8.9 to present all combinations of the two major types of treatment only. Thus the category 'no fillings/no extractions' includes people whose treatment consisted of only a check-up, or a scale and polish or some other form of treatment associated with the health of the soft tissues and those people who had treatment relating to their dentures only.

When asked in 1978 about their most recent course of treatment a smaller proportion of people than in 1968 said they had teeth extracted, the difference being mainly among the group who had extractions only and no fillings. There was, on the other hand, a considerable increase in the group who had neither extractions nor fillings but there had also been some increase in the proportion who had fillings only.

The figures for the different age groups show similar relationships to those seen in the dental examination data with a decrease in extractive treatment for all ages, an increase in conservative treatment among all ages except the youngest age group and an increase in the proportion having neither fillings nor extractions among the younger adults. There was still a greater proportion of older adults than younger adults, however, who had extractions only at their last course of treatment.

Grouping people by their dental attendance pattern (Table 8.10) shows that the large overall reduction in the proportion of people who had extractions and no fillings occurred among the irregular dental attenders while the increase in the proportion having neither fillings, nor extractions was mainly evident among the regular dental attenders. These changes were found in all the regions with the increase in the proportion having no fillings or extractions being greatest among the regular attenders in the Midlands and East Anglia. Although there had been a

Table 8.9 Major type of treatment received at most recent course of treatment for dentate adults in different age groups

Last course of treatment	Age											
	16-24		25-34		35-44		45-54		55 and over		All ages	
	1968	1978	1968	1978	1968	1978	1968	1978	1968	1978	1968	1978
	%	%	%	%	%	%	%	%	%	%	%	%
No fillings/no extractions	20	36	22	34	23	28	24	25	28	33	23	32
Some fillings/no extractions	49	43	36	41	31	39	28	38	18	22	34	37
Some fillings/some extractions	11	8	16	7	11	10	11	9	10	9	12	9
No fillings/some extractions	20	12	26	17	35	23	36	28	44	36	31	22
Don't know	—	1	—	1	—	—	1	—	—	—	—	—
Total	100	100	100	100	100	100	100	100	100	100	100	100
Base	*391*	*634*	*480*	*729*	*429*	*610*	*282*	*454*	*272*	*481*	*1854*	*2912*

Those who were under treatment at the time of the interview have been excluded, as the final extent of the treatment was not known.

decrease for each region in the proportion of irregular attenders who had extractions and no fillings and a corresponding increase in the proportion having only fillings, the proportion who received some conservative treatment at their most recent course of treatment was still highest in London and the South East.

8.5 Overall experience of treatment

We now go on to look briefly at people's overall experiences at the dental surgery in terms of whether they had ever had a filling and, if so, whether they had ever had an injection for a filling and whether they had ever had an X-ray taken of their teeth (Tables 8.11 and 8.12).

Overall, the proportion of adults who had ever had a filling had risen slightly but the figures for the different age groups show that this seemed to be mainly due to the movement through the age structure of the younger people who were more likely to have had fillings. Among those who had had a filling there was also an increase in the proportion who had had an injection. The experience of injections had increased for every age group and within age cohorts suggesting that the use of injections has been increasing over the last ten years.

Given that the dental examination showed very few regular dental attenders to have no fillings it is not particularly surprising to see that nearly all people in this group had experience of having a filling. This was so in 1968 and 1978 and for all parts of the country. The use of injections for fillings, however, does seem to have increased among this group particularly in the North and the Midlands and East Anglia. Among people who only

go to the dentist when they have trouble with their teeth the proportion with experience of fillings had increased from 73% to 79% and of these people the proportion who had ever had an injection had increased substantially from 58% in 1968 to 78% in 1978. The increase in the proportion who had ever had a filling was most marked in Wales and the South West while the increase in the experience of having an injection was largest among irregular dental attenders in the North and London and the South East.

When asked, in 1978, if they had ever had an X-ray taken of their teeth, 59% of dentate adults said they had, compared with 46% in 1968. There was an increase in the experience of having an X-ray both within equivalent age groups and within age cohorts which suggested, as we also saw for the use of injections, that there had been an increase in the use of X-rays over the last ten years. In 1978 three out of four people who go to the dentist for regular check-ups said their teeth had been X-rayed at some time compared with two out of three in 1968. Among those who only go to the dentist when having trouble with their teeth the proportion who had experience of an X-ray had increased substantially from 27% in 1968 to 42% in 1978 suggesting once again that in 1978 this dental attendance group had more experience of long term conservative treatment than they had ten years earlier.

In 1968, we found large regional variations in the use of X-rays in the dental surgery which meant that the treatment of decay was being carried out at different stages in different regions. This was still the case in 1978. Among

Table 8.10 Major type of treatment received at most recent course of treatment by region and dental attendance pattern

Last course of treatment	Those who attend for a regular check-up									
	The North		Wales & the South West		Midlands & East Anglia		London & the South East		England & Wales	
	1968	1978	1968	1978	1968	1978	1968	1978	1968	1978
	%	%	%	%	%	%	%	%	%	%
No fillings/no extractions	45	51	42	47	34	51	36	43	39	47
Some fillings/no extractions	44	41	52	45	60	42	53	49	52	45
Some fillings/some extractions	7	5	—	4	3	4	6	3	5	4
No fillings/some extractions	4	3	6	4	3	3	5	5	4	4
Don't know	—	—	—	—	—	—	—	—	—	—
Total	100	100	100	100	100	100	100	100	100	100
Base	*170*	*260*	*84*	*210*	*155*	*282*	*310*	*408*	*719*	*1160*

Last course of treatment	Those who attend only when having trouble with their teeth									
	The North		Wales & the South West		Midlands & East Anglia		London & the South East		England & Wales	
	1968	1978	1968	1978	1968	1978	1968	1978	1968	1978
	%	%	%	%	%	%	%	%	%	%
No fillings/no extractions	12	15	12	13	12	14	12	15	12	15
Some fillings/no extractions	15	25	13	22	10	14	22	39	16	26
Some fillings/some extractions	18	13	11	18	14	12	20	12	17	13
No fillings/some extractions	55	46	63	47	64	60	45	32	54	45
Don't know	—	1	1	—	—	—	1	2	1	1
Total	100	100	100	100	100	100	100	100	100	100
Base	*254*	*344*	*122*	*186*	*220*	*281*	*326*	*373*	*922*	*1184*

Table 8.11 Experience of fillings and injections among dentate adults in different age groups by region and attendance pattern

		Age					
		16-24	25-34	35-44	45-54	55 and over	All ages
Proportion of dentate adults who had ever had a filling	1968	91% *391*	89% *480*	89% *429*	85% *282*	70% *272*	86% *1854*
	1978	93% *634*	92% *729*	89% *610*	90% *454*	84% *481*	90% *2912*
Proportion* who had ever had injection for a filling	1968	75% *355*	78% *428*	74% *381*	65% *240*	58% *193*	72% *1597*
	1978	86% *585*	91% *666*	89% *540*	83% *406*	76% *401*	86% *2603*

		Those who attend for a regular check-up				
		The North	Wales & the South West	Midlands & East Anglia	London & the South East	England & Wales
Proportion of dentate adults who had ever had a filling	1968	98% *170*	98% *84*	100% *155*	99% *310*	99% *719*
	1978	100% *282*	99% *233*	99% *299*	100% *451*	99% *1265*
Proportion* who had ever had injection for a filling	1968	82% *167*	88% *82*	79% *155*	87% *308*	84% *712*
	1978	91% *281*	92% *232*	90% *295*	92% *449*	91% *1257*

		Those who attend only when having trouble with their teeth				
		The North	Wales & the South West	Midlands & East Anglia	London & the South East	England & Wales
Proportion of dentate adults who had ever had a filling	1968	73% *254*	63% *122*	66% *220*	83% *326*	73% *922*
	1978	76% *357*	82% *192*	68% *288*	89% *393*	79% *1230*
Proportion* who had ever had injection for a filling	1968	50% *185*	69% *77*	58% *144*	62% *272*	58% *678*
	1978	76% *266*	77% *157*	71% *194*	83% *347*	78% *964*

* *Of dentate adults who had ever had a filling*

Table 8.12 Experience of X-rays among dentate adults in different age groups, by region and attendance pattern

		Age					
		16-24	25-34	35-44	45-54	55 and over	All ages
Proportion of dentate adults who had ever had an X-ray	1968	48% *391*	50% *480*	48% *429*	42% *282*	36% *272*	46% *1854*
	1978	61% *634*	66% *729*	62% *610*	55% *454*	44% *481*	59% *2912*

		Those who attend for a regular check-up				
		The North	Wales & the South West	Midlands & East Anglia	London & the South East	England & Wales
Proportion of dentate adults who had ever had an X-ray	1968	54% *170*	64% *84*	57% *155*	81% *310*	67% *719*
	1978	63% *282*	74% *233*	65% *299*	89% *451*	75% *1265*

		Those who attend only when having trouble with their teeth				
		The North	Wales & the South West	Midlands & East Anglia	London & the South East	England & Wales
Proportion of dentate adults who had ever had an X-ray	1968	18% *254*	20% *122*	16% *220*	44% *326*	27% *922*
	1978	34% *123*	36% *192*	24% *288*	64% *393*	42% *1230*

Table 8.13 Whether people had ever been given a demonstration on how to clean their teeth

		Age					
		16-24	25-34	35-44	45-54	55 and over	All ages
Proportion of dentate adults to whom teeth cleaning had been demonstrated	1968	19% *391*	18% *480*	20% *429*	15% *282*	9% *272*	17% *1854*
	1978	29% *634*	31% *729*	30% *610*	28% *454*	21% *481*	28% *2912*

		Those who attend for a regular check-up				
		The North	Wales & the South West	Midlands & East Anglia	London & the South East	England & Wales
Proportion of dentate adults to whom teeth cleaning had been demonstrated	1968	17% *170*	24% *84*	24% *155*	32% *310*	26% *719*
	1978	33% *282*	39% *233*	32% *299*	46% *451*	38% *1265*

		Those who attend only when having trouble with their teeth				
		The North	Wales & the South West	Midlands & East Anglia	London & the South East	England & Wales
Proportion of dentate adults to whom teeth cleaning had been demonstrated	1968	9% *254*	9% *122*	10% *220*	11% *326*	10% *922*
	1978	16% *357*	12% *192*	12% *288*	25% *393*	17% *1230*

both groups of dental attenders the increase in the proportion of people who had ever had an X-ray was similar in each of the regions to that seen overall. This meant that people in London and the South East retained their position of having by far the most experience of the use of X-rays.

In addition to the treatment of dental disease, dentists may also give their patients advice on the care of their teeth. If the number of people who have been given advice increases, then this may lead to a change of attitudes in the general population and may in the long term lead to an improvement in dental health. Both the 1968 and 1978 surveys asked if the informant had ever had toothbrushing demonstrated and Table 8.13 shows that while in 1968 17% had said they had seen a demonstration, in 1978 this proportion had increased to 28%. This increase was apparent for all age groups.

A comparison of the regular dental attenders with those who only attend when they have trouble with their teeth shows that the increase in people receiving a demonstration was larger among the regular attenders of whom more had already said in 1968 that they had seen a demonstration of toothbrushing. This was true for every region apart from London and the South East where the increase in people having toothbrushing demonstrated to them was as large among irregular dental attenders as it was among those who went for regular check-ups. This resulted in a far larger proportion of irregular dental attenders in London and the South East than in other areas who said they had seen a demonstration of toothbrushing.

8.6 The edentulous

So far in this chapter we have been concerned with the changes in attitudes and experiences of dentate adults on the premise that people who still have their own teeth are in a position to maintain or even improve the condition of their natural dentition. This is not so, of course, among the edentulous for whom the irrevocable step has been taken.

However, changes in attitude among those who have lost all their natural teeth may serve to influence the dentate people around them in their determination or otherwise to preserve their natural teeth. One useful indicator of the way people feel about being edentulous is whether or not they are worried about being seen by their family without their dentures (Table 8.14).

Table 8.14 Whether or not people who have lost all their natural teeth mind being seen without their dentures by their family

How much informant is worried about family seeing them without dentures	Male		Female		Both sexes	
	1968	1978	1968	1978	1968	1978
Very much	6	11	15	28	11	21
To some extent	14	11	18	16	16	14
Not at all	70	68	59	49	64	57
No family/ never had denture	10	10	8	7	9	8
Total	100	100	100	100	100	100
Base	455	466	623	696	1078	1162

In 1968, 11% of edentulous people said this worried them very much and by 1978 this proportion had risen to 21%. However, in 1978 there were still 57% of people who said being seen without their dentures did not worry them at all. A greater proportion of women than of men in 1968 said that being seen without their dentures worried them very much. By 1978 this difference had, in fact, increased with 11% of men saying it worried them very much and 28% of women saying this. Thus the results suggest that having no natural teeth is gradually becoming less socially acceptable. If this is the case then individuals may not be so willing to ask their dentist if he will extract all their teeth which is in fact shown in Table 8.15.

Table 8.15 Who suggested the informant became edentulous for people who had lost their teeth in 1958-68 and 1968-78

Who suggested that the last of the natural teeth should be extracted	People who lost the last of their natural teeth in:	
	1958-68	1968-78
	%	%
Informant	41	34
Dentist	50	55
Other	9	11
Total	100	100
Base	295	228

Thus we have seen that the kind of treatment being given has changed over the period of the two surveys and is consistent with the changes in people's attitudes towards, and preferences for conservative treatment as reported earlier in the chapter. It cannot, however, be discerned from the survey whether the treatment provided is influencing people's attitudes, or whether changes in attitudes are affecting treatment, but the results conclusively point towards a dental environment where restorative treatment is now more highly valued than in the past.

Appendix A   The sample

A.1 Introduction

This survey was carried out for the United Kingdom health departments by Social Survey Division in collaboration with the Department of Dental Health, University of Birmingham Dental School. Previous surveys of adult dental health had been carried out in England and Wales in 1968, and in Scotland in 1972. A survey of children's dental health in England and Wales had been undertaken in 1973.

The aim of the survey was to discover the state of individuals' dental health and to ask about their dental experiences in order to help plan and organise the dental services in the future. Comparison with past data would indicate whether or not dental health was improving.

Since the survey was intended to provide data for comparison with the results of the previous work the data collected and analyses undertaken had to be essentially the same as before. However, in 1974 the National Health Service had been reorganised and it was considered important for any regional analysis to be relevant to the current organisation of the provision of dental services.

The main change in the overall scheme was that only people with some natural teeth were to have a dental examination although all people were to be interviewed.

A.2 Population

The population concerned was that of adults (ie those aged 16 and over) throughout the United Kingdom. Scotland and Wales were oversampled so that some separate analyses could be carried out in those areas, but Northern Ireland was included proportionately for the purpose of providing total figures for the UK.

A.3 Sample size and expected precision

One of the main determinants of sample size in this survey was the need to be able to detect any major changes that had occurred in the dental health of adults in England and Wales between 1968 and 1978. We also wished to detect major changes in the dental condition of adults in Scotland, but, because of the shorter time period between the previous Scottish survey and the 1978 survey, less detailed analyses were planned.

An important indicator of the dental condition of a population is the proportion who have no natural teeth. It is possible to calculate the probability of detecting a given difference between two percentages at the 5% level of significance (see W G Cochran and G M Cox *Experimental Designs* 1966).

The previous surveys had estimates of the proportion edentulous in England and Wales and in Scotland. We also knew from various sources the estimated size of the proportion edentulous for 1978 and so we were able to use these figures to determine the sample size.

i) England and Wales

In order to detect a true decrease of 6% between 37% (edentulous 1968) and 31% (expected edentulous 1978*) at the 5% level of significance, with level of certainty P, the following achieved sample sizes (n) are required:

P	n
53%	370
64%	500
71%	600
76%	700

ii) Scotland

Similarly, in order to detect a true decrease of 3% between 44% (edentulous 1972) and 41% (expected edentulous 1978*) at the 5% level of significance, with level of certainty P, the following achieved sample sizes (n) are required:

P	n
31%	700
44%	1200
50%	1500
60%	1960

A constraint was imposed on the sample size for this survey by the number of dentists available for carrying out examinations and the fact that each dentist required a workload which was contained in a clearly defined area and involved the minimum of travelling time. This effectively restricted the number of primary sampling units which could be used.

In view of these considerations, it was decided to select a sample of 7,500 in which Scotland was weighted by 3.3 and Wales by 2.4.

A.4 Effect of weighting

Before carrying out the survey it was possible to consider the effect of weighting on the variance of estimates. The expected increase in the variance was calculated using:

$$V^2 = W_h K_h \left(\sum \frac{W_h}{K_h} \right) \frac{S^2}{N}$$

(L Kish *Survey Sampling*, 1965)

---

* Figure obtained from a survey carried out in 1977 by Market and Opinion Research International

where W_h = $\dfrac{\text{total population in stratum h}}{\text{total population in all strata}}$

K_h = weight to be applied in stratum

S = variance of an estimate

N = sample size

Calculations showed that when Scotland was weighted by 3.3 and Wales by 2.4, the variance of an estimate would be increased by a factor of 1.6.

A.5 Sub-groups

The estimates of precision presented in 'sample size and expected precision' above assumed the analysis of the whole sample, whereas the analysis of subgroups is an important consideration. In particular, the dentate in the sample form an important group and Table A.1 shows the expected numbers of these people and of those who would be examined by dentists (assuming 90% response to examination).

Clearly, the precision of estimates for this subgroup (the dentate) would be lower than for the whole sample. For example, taking 37% as an estimate of the proportion of regular dental attenders among the dentate in Wales in 1968* we would be able to detect an increase of 5% with only 39% certainty.

Table A.1 Expected number of dentate in sample

	Achieved sample	Expected dentate	Exams achieved (90% response)
Scotland	1526 x0.59	900	810
Wales	588 x0.61	359	323
Northern Ireland	137 x0.61	84	76
England	4124 x0.69	2846	2561
Northern & Yorks	595	411	370
Mersey & North West	584	403	363
Trent & East Anglia	562	388	349
West Midlands	460	317	285
South Western, Wessex & Oxford	710	490	441
NE & NW Thames	638	440	396
SE & SW Thames	575	397	357
United Kingdom	**6375**	**4189**	**3770**

A.6 Sample design

It is generally accepted that for any ratio estimate to have an acceptably low maximum bias at least 40 primary sampling units (50 to be certain) are necessary. This applies to any level of analysis (regional, etc.) but practical constraints meant that we could only follow this guideline for estimates relating to England and Wales combined.

Since the number of PSUs was relatively small it was considered advisable to use a two-stage rather than three-stage design to overcome the effects of clustering. Constituencies were chosen as first stage units because this would result in the areas to be covered by both dentists and interviewers being smaller in many parts of the country than if another unit (such as District) were used, but also in the sample being less clustered than if wards were used.

---

* In the 1968 survey, it was found that in Wales and the South West 43% of those aged 16-34 and 30% of those aged 35 or more who were dentate attended a dentist regularly.

Table A.2 Distribution of a sample of 7,500 (Scotland weighted by 3.3 Wales by 2.4)

	Set sample		Expected achieved sample (85% response)
	Individuals	Constituencies	
Scotland	1795	20	1526
Wales	692	12	588
Northern Ireland	161	2	137
England	4852	39	4124
Northern & Yorks	700	6	595
Mersey & North West	687	6	584
Trent & East Anglia	661	5	562
West Midlands	541	4	460
South Western, Wessex & Oxford	835	7	710
NE & NW Thames	751	6	638
SE & SW Thames	677	5	575
United Kingdom	**7500**	**73**	**6375**

The regions to be used for analysis were formed by grouping adjacent Regional Health Authorities. Table A.2 shows the distribution of the set and expected achieved sample.

Distribution of the sample between regions was carried out with probability proportional to the 1975 population (the most recent figures available). Constituencies were selected with probability proportional to 1977 electorate.

With an achieved sample of the size shown in Tables A.1 and A.2, we would be more than 50% certain of detecting the expected change in Scotland, and 89% certain of detecting the expected change in the smallest regional group to be used in the comparative study. (The Midlands and East Anglia which was equivalent to the grouped Regional Health Authorities of West Midlands, Trent and East Anglia.)

A.7 Stratification

Four stratification factors relevant to the survey were used:

i) Region: Scotland, Wales and Northern Ireland formed one region each and England was divided into the seven grouped Regional Health Authority regions shown in the tables. (Within region, Scottish constituencies were also stratified according to whether they were city, highland and island, or other type.)

ii) Socio-Economic Group: Constituencies were ordered by the proportion of the population in SEG 1 to 5 and 13.

iii) Age: For each constituency the proportion of the population aged 60 years or more was calculated using census data (age being related to tooth loss).

iv) Persons Per Dentist (1976): The Dental Estimates Board produces these figures for counties and Family Practitioner Committee Areas. Constituencies in England and Wales were allocated the appropriate value for the area in which they fell. (Figures were not available for Scotland or Northern Ireland).

A.8 Regional comparisons with the 1968 survey

The eight regions of England and Wales used in the design of the sample were formed by geographically grouping Regional Health Authorities. However, the 1968 survey of England and Wales, with which comparisons were to be made, had been analysed in terms of grouped planning regions which were not wholly contiguous with Health Authorities. This meant that it was not possible simply to regroup the eight RHA regions in order to obtain the equivalent of the four grouped planning region areas.

It was suggested that each constituency might be reallocated to one of the four 1968 regions at the analysis stage. Since the sample was stratified by RHA region, this may have meant that it was unrepresentative in a particular region, and therefore, any estimate biased. However, as the two sets of regions overlap to the greater extent and the grouped planning regions are larger than the RHA regions, the problem should be negligible.

A.9 Large constituencies

When the sample of constituencies had been drawn, it became apparent that some of them covered too large an area for one dental examiner to cover adequately. It was therefore decided that the sample design should be subject to a further stage in those nine constituencies which covered more than 250,000 acres. In these cases, grouped wards were selected with probability proportional to 1977 electorate.

A.10 Sample selection of individuals

Since the population of interest was that of adults aged 16 and over, and because the Electoral Register covers only those aged 18 and over the sampling method used had to include the selection of the correct proportion of 16 and 17 year olds and, also, any other people who happened not to be registered. The Marchant and Blyth Method of selecting individuals fulfills both these criteria and so was used in the selection of the sample. (See Annex to this sampling report). The inclusion of 16 and 17 year olds also had to be allowed for in the initial planning of the numbers of people to be selected so that the sample size would reach 7,500 after the inclusion of the selected 16 and 17 year olds.

The distribution of the selected sample is shown in Table A.3.

In Scottish cities the procedure was somewhat different from elsewhere. When four or more surnames were registered at an address, we took a household, rather than the address, as the unit of interest. Thus, on the address form, we listed the selected person and anyone else at the address with the same surname (surnames being taken as an approximation to households) while everyone else at the address was included on a supplementary list. In these cases, interviewers were instructed to list on the address form only additional members of the selected person's household (rather than address) and then to check whether any of these had been included on the supplementary list. If this was the case, the person in question was deleted from the address form in such a way as to make it clear what had happened. This meant that, when the address form was returned to the office, any additional interviews carried out in the household could be reweighted if they had initially been given the wrong chance of selection. In the event this occurred in only two cases so it was agreed that reweighting the data for two individuals would introduce unnecessary complications in the analysis.

A.11 Northern Ireland

It was agreed that the Department of Finance, on behalf of the Department of Health and Social Services in Northern Ireland, should select its own sample of four districts and two wards within each, from a frame stratified by population density only. The total number of individuals selected was to be that calculated by Sampling Branch of Social Survey Division.

A.12 Response

Table A.4 shows the overall response figures. The number of individuals selected throughout the UK was 7266. However, it was apparent from the Electoral Register that 113 of the addresses involved were institutions of some kind (for example, old people's homes, university halls of residence, etc.) and as institutions were to be excluded from the sample, these were withdrawn before the addresses were allocated to interviewers, leaving a sample of 7153.

When interviewers tried to make contact at these addresses, they found 878 cases where an interview was not required because the address no longer existed, it was

Table A.3 The selected sample

	Estimated sample size	No. of constituencies	Sample per constituency	Actual sample size
Scotland	1732	20	87	1740
Wales	668	12	56	672
Northern Ireland	155	2*	78*	156*
England	4682	39	120	4680
Northern & Yorks	676	6	113	678
Mersey & North West	663	6	111	666
Trent & East Anglia	638	5	128	640
West Midlands	522	4	131	524
South Western, Wessex and Oxford	806	7	115	805
NE & NW Thames	725	6	121	726
SE & SW Thames	653	5	131	655
United Kingdom	**7237**	**73**		**7262**

* In Northern Ireland 160 individuals were actually selected (see above).

empty, or the selected person had moved away and insufficient people had moved in for another person to be selected.

The number of addresses lost at this stage was slightly higher than we expected which was probably due to the age of the Electoral Register used to select the sample. In 1968 the fieldwork dates were chosen to allow the interviewing to start as soon as practically possible after the compilation of the Electoral Register. In order to reduce losses from the sample due to changes in address occurring between the time people were registered and when the interviewer went to interview them. However, in 1978, the exclusion of the edentulous from the examination meant that, while keeping the size of the dental team reasonably small, we were able to select a larger sample overall. Since we were dealing with a much larger sample it was necessary to begin the selection procedure earlier which meant that the sample could not be selected from the new Electoral Register as had been the case in 1968. Thus in 1978 there was a year longer between people registering and the interviewers going to the address in which changes, such as people moving or property being demolished, could have occurred.

Table A.4 Response

a)	Sample of address	
	Number of addresses selected	7266
	Withdrawn (obvious institutions)	113
	Set sample	7153
	No person for interview at address	878
	Effective sample	6275
b)	Co-operation achieved at the interview	
	Interview obtained	5967
	Refusal	529
	Non-contact	183
	Total people selected from 6,275 address	6679

At the addresses in the effective sample, a total of 6679 eligible people were present. Of these, 712 either refused to be interviewed or could not be contacted by the interviewer and the remaining 5967 agreed to participate.

It had been anticipated that over 240 people aged 16 or 17 would be selected by interviewers and interviewed.

However, only 146 of this group were included*. There are several possible explanations for this: firstly it may be that 16 and 17 year olds were less easy to contact and produced a higher level of non-response than the sample as a whole, secondly, interviewers may not have made it clear that they were interested in contacting people of this age, and thirdly, this group may not always have come within the standard household definition used because they were away at school or college.

A.13 Comparison of the sample with the population
The characteristics of the achieved sample were compared with those of the population of the UK in order to find whether the sample was representative.

The distribution of individuals between the grouped Regional Health Authorities was not significantly different from that of those aged 16 years and over in the population. However, when regrouping into standard regions was carried out for comparison with the 1968 data, Wales and the South West was found to contain too large a proportion of the sample.

Neither the sex nor age structure of the sample showed any significant differences for the UK as a whole, although some individual countries and regions were not completely representative. In the case of sex, South Western, Wessex and Oxford had slightly fewer men in the sample than would be expected, but no other regions or countries showed any differences. With regard to age, the sample was deficient in 16 to 24 year olds in England, and that country also had too low a proportion of those aged 75 or over and too high a proportion of 35 to 44 year olds (Table A.5). Looking again at the total sample, it was deficient in women aged 75 or over and men aged 16 to 34, and contained too large a proportion of men aged 35 to 44.

Comparison of the age structure of the sample within grouped Regional Health Authorities was difficult as the figures available included 15 year olds in the youngest age

---

* There were 146 people interviewed who said that they were aged 16 or 17 years on 1 May 1978, but interviewers were instructed to establish eligibility by means of age at time of first contact.

Table A.5 Comparison of sample and population age and sex distributions by country

Age/Sex	England		Scotland		Wales		UK	
	Weighted achieved sample	Population estimate	Weighted achieved sample	Population estimate	Weighted achieved sample	Population estimate	Weighted achieved sample	Population estimate
	%	%	%	%	%	%	%	%
16-24	16	17	17	19	13	17	16	18
25-34	18	19	19	18	19	18	18	18
35-44	17	15	17	15	18	15	17	15
45-54	16	15	16	15	16	15	16	15
55-64	15	15	15	14	17	15	15	15
65-74	12	12	10	12	12	13	12	12
75 and over	6	7	6	7	5	7	6	7
	100	100	100	100	100	100	100	100
Male	47	49	47	48	47	49	47	48
Female	53	51	53	52	53	51	53	52
	100	100	100	100	100	100	100	100
Base	*3833*	*35,586,000*	*1420*	*3,928,000*	*580*	*2,132,000*	*4639*	*42,728,000*

group. However, bearing this in mind, it appeared that four regions (Northern & Yorks, Mersey & North West, West Midlands, and South Western Wessex and Oxford) were deficient in the youngest age group (16 to 24) and North Thames was unusual in having an excess. We also found that West Midlands had too few 25 to 34 year olds while Mersey & North West, West Midlands and South Thames all had an excess of 35 to 44 year olds and Mersey and North West and North Thames both had too few of those aged 75 years and over.

A.14 Sampling errors
The variance of a population variable assuming simple random sampling can be estimated from the sample using:

$$s^2 = \sum_{i=1}^{n} \frac{(y_i - \bar{y})^2}{n-1}$$

Where n = the number of elements in the sample each with value y_i and $\bar{y}$ = the mean of these values.
The estimated variance of an estimate of the mean value of y in the population depends on the number of observations that make up the sample and is given by:

$$\text{variance } (\bar{y}) = \frac{s^2}{n}$$

However, calculations based on the above formulae do not take into account the two-stage design or the stratification used in the sample design of this survey. Kish and Hess[1] describe a means of estimating the error due to the multi-stage sample based only on the sample variance between first stage units.

The 75 first stage units were selected systematically within regions from lists ordered by the stratification factors. This type of design can be regarded as the selection of one unit from each of a number of 'implicit' strata. In order to calculate the variance it is necessary to 'collapse' adjacent strata so that in our calculations we have two first stage units per stratum.

All possible adjacent pairings are made within region so that 1 is compared with 2, 2 with 3, 3 with 4 and so on until the end of the region. Thus the calculations are based on $L_h - 1$ differences where L_h is the number of PSU's selected from region h.

The formula is given for the ratio estimator $r = y/x$ where x_i, y_i are values for two variables for the ith informant and x, y are the sums of these variables.

The estimated variance of r is given by:

$$\hat{var}(r) = \frac{1}{x^2} \sum_{h=1}^{H} \frac{L_h}{2(L_h-1)} \left[\sum_{\alpha=1}^{L_h-1} dy_{h\alpha}^2 + r^2 \sum_{\alpha=1}^{L_h-1} dx_{h\alpha}^2 \right.$$
$$\left. -2r \sum_{\alpha=1}^{L_h-1} dy_{h\alpha} \, dx_{h\alpha} \right]$$

Where
L is the number of strata

$$dy_{h\alpha} = y_{h\alpha} - y_{h\alpha+1}$$
$$dx_{h\alpha} = x_{h\alpha} - x_{h\alpha+1}$$

$x_{h\alpha}$ and $y_{h\alpha}$ are weighed totals of the x and y variables from stratum $h\alpha$.

This formula is only valid where the coefficient of variation of x, $cv(x)$ is small. Kish[1] recommends that ideally $cv(x)$ should be less than 0.1 and should definitely be below 0.2 for the approximation to be reasonable. We examined the coefficient of variation for each of the variables for which we calculated the variances. The majority were smaller than 0.1 and none were greater than 0.2.

Sampling errors based on the above formula are presenteed for a selection of the survey variables and subgroups in the following tables. Also shown are the values of the simple random errors and the square root of the design effect. The design effect ('deff') is the ratio of the variance of a statistic, calculated taking into account the two-stage design, to the variance of the same statistic based on a simple random sample of the same size. Thus the square root of deff is the multiple that needs to be applied to the estimated simple random sampling error to take account of the complex design. The variance of multi-stage samples is generally greater than for a comparable single stage sample and so $\sqrt{deff}$ is usually larger than one.

The values of $\sqrt{deff}$ presented in the following tables range from 0.75 to 2.6 for the data and 0.88 to 2.0 for the 1968 data. Most values fell between 0.9 and 1.3 for both surveys with the 1968 values being slightly lower in general than those for 1978. This was probably due to the 1978 sample not being self-weighting.

The largest design effects were found in the decay measures. This might be expected since the complex error calculation is based on the differences between primary sampling units and each dental examiner worked wholly within one or two primary sampling units. Thus we are effectively taking account of the differences between dental examiners and of all the different tooth conditions the measurement of decay showed the greatest variability during the calibration exercise.

A.15 Comparing two statistics
Frequently we wish to examine the difference between two statistics such as the proportion of edentulous men and the proportion of edentulous women. The difference between two ratios $(r - r^l)$ has a variance which is estimated by:

$$\text{var} (r - r^l) = \text{var} (r) + \text{var} (r^l) - 2 \text{ covariance} (r \, r^l)$$

Since the 1968 survey and the 1978 survey were conducted on difference samples the covariance of their results is zero. Therefore when comparisons are made between the

Table A.6 Sampling errors of the percentage edentulous (UK 1978)*

Sex/Age	Base sample size	Percentage edentulous	Sampling error		√deff
			Simple random	Complex	
Male	2176	25.4	0.95	0.93	0.98
Female	2463	33.4	0.95	1.15	1.21
16-24	729	0.4	0.24	0.18	0.75
45-54	728	31.5	1.72	1.68	0.98
65 and over	821	79.1	1.42	1.50	1.06
United Kingdom	**4639**	**29.7**	**0.67**	**0.86**	**1.28**

* In 1978 the analysis of the survey data was based on two different areas: the United Kingdom and England and Wales. Initial investigations showed that complex sampling errors for variables and sub-groups based on England and Wales data were about 1.1 times as large as those for the same variables and sub-groups based on UK data. Since it was impracticable to produce both sets of errors for all sub-groups and variables we present the 1978 sampling errors for the United Kingdom sample.

Table A.7 Sampling errors of the percentage edentulous (England and Wales 1968)*

Sex/Age	Base sample size	Percentage edentulous	Sampling error		√deff
			Simple random	Complex	
Male	1382	33.0	1.26	1.43	1.13
Female	1550	40.2	1.24	1.43	1.15
16-24	395	1.0	0.50	0.46	0.92
45-54	475	40.6	2.25	2.22	0.99
65 and over	503	81.7	1.72	1.68	0.98
England and Wales	**2932**	**36.8**	**0.89**	**1.04**	**1.17**

Table A.8 Sampling errors for mean tooth conditions (UK 1978 - people with some natural teeth)

Category	Base sample size	Mean no. of teeth	Sampling error		√deff
			Simple random	Complex	
Missing teeth					
Male	1396	9.1	0.20	0.23	1.15
Female	1387	8.8	0.18	0.18	1.00
16-24	646	4.9	0.12	0.12	1.00
45-54	419	12.6	0.32	0.38	1.19
Regular attender	1267	7.6	0.15	0.15	1.00
Only with trouble	1114	10.9	0.25	0.28	1.12
United Kingdom	**2783**	**9.0**	**0.13**	**0.14**	**1.08**
Sound teeth					
Male	1396	13.3	0.18	0.23	1.28
Female	1387	12.7	0.17	0.19	1.12
16-24	646	17.1	0.23	0.24	1.04
45-54	419	10.4	0.26	0.28	1.08
Regular attender	1267	11.9	0.15	0.17	1.13
Only with trouble	1114	13.7	0.22	0.27	1.23
United Kingdom	**2783**	**13.0**	**0.12**	**0.16**	**1.33**
Filled (otherwise sound) teeth					
Male	1396	7.3	0.16	0.17	1.06
Female	1387	8.9	0.16	0.20	1.25
16-24	646	8.0	0.21	0.26	1.24
45-54	419	7.1	0.27	0.32	1.18
Regular attender	1267	11.4	0.14	0.17	1.21
Only with trouble	1114	4.4	0.15	0.17	1.13
United Kingdom	**2783**	**8.1**	**0.11**	**0.16**	**1.45**
Decayed teeth					
Male	1396	2.2	0.08	0.15	1.88
Female	1387	1.6	0.07	0.13	1.86
16-24	646	2.0	0.12	0.22	1.83
45-54	419	1.9	0.13	0.16	1.23
Regular attender	1267	1.1	0.05	0.13	2.60
Only with trouble	1114	3.0	0.11	0.18	1.64
United Kingdom	**2783**	**1.9**	**0.05**	**0.13**	**2.60**

Table A.9 Sampling errors for mean tooth conditions (England and Wales 1968 - people with some natural teeth)

Category	Base sample size	Mean no. of teeth	Sampling error		√deff
			Simple random	Complex	
Missing teeth					
Male	858	9.8	0.24	0.21	0.88
Female	836	10.3	0.25	0.25	1.00
16-24	371	5.2	0.16	0.16	1.00
45-54	257	14.5	0.44	0.42	0.95
Regular attender	680	7.8	0.21	0.21	1.00
Only with trouble	817	12.4	0.27	0.26	0.96
England & Wales	**1694**	**10.0**	**0.17**	**0.15**	**0.88**
Sound teeth					
Male	858	13.3	0.22	0.24	1.09
Female	836	12.3	0.20	0.23	1.15
16-24	371	16.4	0.27	0.27	1.00
45-54	257	10.3	0.33	0.35	1.06
Regular attender	680	11.8	0.19	0.22	1.16
Only with trouble	817	13.4	0.24	0.26	1.08
England & Wales	**1694**	**12.8**	**0.15**	**0.19**	**1.27**
Filled (otherwise sound) teeth					
Male	858	6.2	0.20	0.26	1.30
Female	836	7.5	0.21	0.24	1.14
16-24	371	8.2	0.30	0.39	1.30
45-54	257	5.0	0.32	0.30	0.94
Regular attender	680	11.1	0.19	0.25	1.32
Only with trouble	817	3.0	0.14	0.17	1.21
England & Wales	**1694**	**6.8**	**0.14**	**0.21**	**1.50**
Decayed teeth					
Male	858	2.6	0.11	0.15	1.36
Female	836	1.8	0.09	0.11	1.22
16-24	371	2.1	0.14	0.23	1.64
45-54	257	2.2	0.18	0.18	1.00
Regular attender	680	1.1	0.06	0.12	2.00
Only with trouble	817	3.2	0.12	0.14	1.17
England & Wales	**1694**	**2.2**	**0.07**	**0.12**	**1.71**

two sets of results the error of the difference is simply the square root of the sum of the two variances.

For comparisons made within the 1978 survey data, however, there will be some measure of covariance. It is possible to calculate the complex sampling error of the difference between two statistics using the Kish and Hess method already described. A selection of these errors is shown in Table A.10.

Throughout the text where two figures are stated to be different from each other this difference has been tested and found to be statistically significant at the 5% level (ie the difference/estimate of complex error of difference ≥ 1.96).

Reference
[1] L Kish & I Hess. On variances of ratios and their differences in multi-stage samples. *Journal of the American Statistical Association* **54** 1959.

Table A.10 Sampling errors of the differences between two statistics (UK 1978)

	Male — female		Regular — only with trouble	
	Difference	Complex error	Difference	Complex error
Percentage edentulous	—8.0	1.22	—	—
Mean number of:				
Missing teeth	0.3	0.30	—3.3	0.31
Sound teeth	0.6	0.26	—1.8	0.32
Filled (otherwise sound) teeth	—1.6	0.21	8.0	0.22
Decayed teeth	0.6	0.09	—1.9	0.12

Annex to sampling report

A note on the Marchant and Blyth Self-weighting random sampling technique

This method of sampling involves a slightly different procedure from that usually employed once the primary sampling units (in this case constituencies) have been selected. A systematic sample of electors is drawn, using the Electoral Register as a frame, and the addresses at which they are registered become the sampling units for the next stage of the procedure.

At this point the method begins to differ from others. Electors are listed at the address in the order in which they appear on the Electoral Register and numbers 1 to 4, spaced at regular intervals, are written down the right hand side of the address form. Number 1 is written next to the name of the elector who led to the selection of the address, and the others are spaced at regular intervals corresponding to the number of electors at the address. The inter-

viewer calls at the sampled address and interviews the selected individual if present. She then lists systematically anyone else living at that address and not already on the list. If any of these additional people fall on numbered lines they are eligible for interview.

This procedure results in all informants having the same chance of selection. At an address with n electors registered, lines 1 to n contain their names and lines $n + 1$ onwards bear those of non-electors. If the elector on line 1 happens to have been the person initially selected then non-electors on lines $n + 1$, $2n + 1$ and so on will also be selected. Hence, all have the same chance of selection, and since within each country all electors at all addresses were originally given the same chance of selection, all informants have the same chance and the sample is self-weighting.

Appendix B

The criteria for clinical assessments, the conduct of the dental examination and the training of examiners

R J Anderson, J H Nunn, P S Hull and
P M C James

Department of Dental Health, University of
Birmingham

United Kingdom Adult Dental Health Survey 1978

Training of dental examiners

Introduction

In an epidemiological exercise on this scale, there is ever present the dilema of either undertaking large numbers of examinations using a small number of examiners, with the risk of a change in the diagnostic criteria because of the extended time scale; or alternatively, of utilising a large number of examiners over as short an examination period as possible with all the attendant problems of examiner variability. As with the earlier national dental studies it was decided to opt for a large dental team and a relatively short field period. This of course meant that the problem of training and standardising a large team had to be faced. However, it was felt for reasons already stated in the main introduction that varying training patterns and differing levels of experience among the team resulting in variability of diagnosis, could be reduced to a minimum by laying down precisely, the criteria for examination, followed by an intensive period of training. This would ensure, as far as possible, that when differences arose in the results, these would be real and not due to individual examiner variation.

In order to obtain as good a response as possible, the dental examination was carried out in people's homes rather than in a centre to which the participants would have had to travel. Of necessity therefore, the scope of the examination was limited to that amount of information that could be readily collected by a dentist using a small amount of mobile equipment and by the amount of time available to undertake such an examination. It was acknowledged that these constraints would necessarily result in some understatement of the true disease levels but that this sacrifice was necessary in order to guarantee meaningful and valid results.

Setting the criteria

The type and extent of the clinical information to be collected was decided upon by a steering committee consisting of representatives of the Department of Health and Social Security, the Office of Population Censuses and Surveys, a dentist from each of the countries involved in the study and members of the Department of Dental Health, the University of Birmingham. Thereafter, discussions and testing of the resultant criteria were carried out by members of the Department of Dental Health in conjunction with the study organisers from the Office of Population Censuses and Surveys (OPCS). The outcome of these deliberations were the criteria that were to be validated at the pre-pilot study. It was important that the sensitivity and specificity of the criteria were such as to detect variation where it truly existed but not so refined as to result in major intra- or inter-examiner variability. The development of the criteria was done in the full awareness that some degree of accuracy would be sacrificed in order to ensure standardisation in data collection.

A further factor in the criteria design was the necessity to retain, as far as was possible, comparison with the England and Wales Adult Dental Health Survey, undertaken in 1968, so that results from both surveys could, where appropriate, be compared.

Pre-pilot study

This was carried out in the autumn of 1977 in the Birmingham Dental Hospital, using technical staff as subjects and members of the Department of Dental Health as examiners, in order to test the feasability of the proposed criteria and methods of data collection. During this time the examination aids, examination charts and diagnostic criteria were thoroughly tested, after modifications, and in conjunction with the members of OPCS criteria and examination charts were drawn up for further field testing in the pilot.

Pilot study

The revised criteria and procedures were further tested in January 1978 by members of the Department of Dental Health together with four area dental officers from different parts of the country. The seven examiners underwent the standardisation and calibration exercise provisionally planned for the main examiner training courses. Analysis of the calibration exercise revealed there to be no major discrepancies in standardisation. At this stage further minor amendments were made to the criteria and the sequence of the examination procedure.

Following the pilot dental training course the examiners undertook to test the criteria and examination techniques further by conducting examinations on members of the public in six pilot areas of the country, with one examiner acting as a reserve.

Main training programme

The 64 dentists who had been seconded to the study met as two separate groups on consecutive weeks in April 1978. Each examiner had been asked to supply certain of the items necessary for the dental examination (listed in Annex 1) the remaining items were issued to them on their arrival. The three instructors for the training programme were members of the Department of Dental Health, University of Birmingham; the more senior of these had been closely involved in the early development work and, together with the other two, had acted as a trainer on the pilot study as well as participating in the field work that followed it. They were assisted in their role, as trainers, by the four area dental officers who had taken part in the pilot work and who now acted as tutors each with responsibility for a group of dentists. In addition, a team from OPCS was present for the second stage of the training programme to monitor and record the results of the practical training sessions. Other members of.OPCS and the Department of Dental Health acted in a supervisory and monitoring role for the duration of the training exercise.

During the introductory period much emphasis was placed on the necessity for the survey examination criteria to take precedence over those used elsewhere in order to ensure complete reproducibility in recording. Furthermore, the concensus arrived at by the examiners, without influence from individual interpretations, during the first training week, was used as a basis for the training of the second group of examiners after slight modifications to the criteria where necessary.

The training programme was divided into three distinct stages; the first part atempted to familiarise the examiners with the criteria, their appropriate codes and the examination chart. This was achieved by short didactic sessions followed by practical work on models and slides of widely varying clinical conditions. After the first day and a half of intensive training, the examiners were taken to an industrial research establishment where members of the staff had agreed to act as subjects for the purposes of examiner training.

In the first half of the first session, the dentists worked in pairs with one acting as a subject and the other as an examiner whilst the tutors took the role of recorders. This period enabled the dentists to familiarise themselves with the application of the criteria to 'real' subjects as opposed to the models and slides, before they were confronted with the volunteer subjects who arrived for the second half of the session at which point the pairs of dentists then took the roles of recorder and examiner. After examining a subject, the two dentists would reverse their roles for the next subject, so that each had experience of examining as well as recording. It was pointed out to them that when taking the part of the recorder they were to carry out the function ascribed without undue recourse to checking the statements of the examiner or conferring on a point of doubt. The emphasis at this stage of the training was on correct procedure and completion of the examination chart without undue pressure on the examiner. On the subsequent two days the same arrangements held for examiner and recorder at these sessions, each examination chart was checked by OPCS staff and compared with the other charts which referred to the same subject as part of the standardisation exercise. This allowed for a constant feed-back of information to the tutors, so that when discrepancies arose they were able to rapidly communicate them to the examiner or examiners involved. On occasion this was done with reference to the subject if he was still present, thereby enabling the original decision to be either confirmed or refuted. It was important at this stage for the tutor to decide if the problem was a serious one and at the same time to elicit whether it was the examiner or the subject that was causing the difficulty, ie was there dispute because of a 'marginal' mouth or a 'marginal' examiner. At the same time, increasing

pressure was put on the examiner to speed up; this was necessary in order that sufficient time would be available to carry out the calibration exercise at the end of the training week.

On the Monday, Tuesday and Wednesday evenings the examiners met with their group tutors informally, with their examination charts in order to discuss any problems that may have arisen that day. If necessary, the models and slides were available so that errors in interpretation or misunderstanding could be discussed. At these meetings attention was also drawn to the way in which a dentist's scores may have differed from those of the rest of the group and the possible reasons why. In this way it was hoped that greater standardisation would be achieved.

Calibration and recalibration
On the last day of the training week the examiners met up with one of the OPCS interviewers with whom they would be working for the forthcoming few weeks. One half of the dentists and interviewers then left for the research establishment where they were to undertake the calibration exercise. For a short period they spent some time looking through the forms which the dentist had collected during the week and callilng from them so that the interviewer could become familiar with any idiosyncracies in calling of codes that her particular dentist may have had. There then followed the calibration exercise in which two groups of eight dentists each saw the same eight subjects, as a means of measuring the differences that might still exist between the examiners. Meanwhile the remaining sixteen dentists and their interviewers also worked through their previously accumulated examination charts. These dentists then took part in the second calibration exercise with a different group of subjects from those examined in the morning. The calibration exercise was carried out in the same way as the standardisation exercises of the previous three days except that this time no attempt was made to check the completed forms of the examiners, at this stage, and the interviewers rather than dentists acted as recorders.

This exercise was repeated at the end of the field work in June 1978, when the two groups of dentists returned to re-examine the same subjects that they had seen at the end of their training week. It was therefore possible to detect any shifts in diagnostic standards, away from the set criteria, that might have occurred during the main field work. Two of the dentists who had been to the original calibration exercise did not conduct any survey examinations and so did not return for the recalibration and, unfortunately, eight of the original volunteer subjects were unable to take part in the recalibration. In order to make comparisons between the two sessions, results have been presented only from those who had been present at both.

Results of calibration and recalibration exercises
Once the results from the calibration and recalibration exercises had been collected certain variables were selected in order to investigate the examiner variation. The selected variables can be divided under three head-

ings — tooth conditions, tooth positions and gum conditions. Within each calibration and recalibration group the total mean value per dentist, for each of the selected variables was calculated together with the standard deviation and the coefficient of variation.

Table B.1 shows these results for the different tooth conditions. The conditions listed are not independent of each other, in that the measurements of 'filled and decayed teeth' and 'decayed, not previously treated, teeth' are the components of the measurement of 'all decayed teeth'. Of the different tooth conditions, the main measures used in the text of this report are the number missing, the total number decayed and the number filled (otherwise sound).

The table shows that the coefficient of variation of the measurement of missing teeth was very low and there was virtually no difference between the number of missing teeth recorded at the calibration session and the recalibration session. The variability of numbers of teeth which were recorded as both filled and decayed was high while the variability of the measurement of filled (otherwise sound) teeth was low.

The results show that detecting the presence of decay gave rise to more variability than for missing or filled teeth and this was so both in the case of decayed and filled teeth and teeth which were decayed and previously untreated. This high variation in measurement occurred at both the calibration and recalibration sessions. It is interesting to note that at the recalibration session, the dentists consistently recorded a lower level of decay than they had previously, there was also generally slightly more variation among the dentists in the recording of teeth which were decayed and previously untreated at the recalibration session than at the calibration session.

Table B.2 shows the variability in the measurements of tooth position, that is whether or not there was a space where a tooth was missing and whether the teeth in a segment were crowded. The coefficients of variation associated with spaces and non-spaces were generally low, though groups two and seven had a slightly higher variability in the measures of both these conditions at both the calibration and recalibration session. In both of these groups there was one dentist who tended to record a high number of spaces and a high number of non-spaces, compared with the other dentists in their groups.

The measurement of crowding showed a higher variability for all the groups of dentists for both calibration and recalibration than the other tooth position measures had shown, though, for most groups, there was more variability in the measurements at the recalibration session than at the calibration session. As has been found in the previous dental surveys the measurement of gum conditions once again proved to be associated with a high level of variability (Table B.3).

Of the four gum conditions measured, gingivitis and calculus showed the lowest coefficients of variation. In most cases, the coefficients were larger for the recalibration results.

There was little periodontitis found among the volunteer subjects and the measurement of it gave rise to high coefficients of variation among nearly all groups of dentists, for both the calibration and recalibration.

For the measurements of debris, the coefficients of variation were similar at the calibration and recalibration (except in the case of group seven where there was a much higher coefficient of variation for the recalibration results than for the calibration results). The estimation of the amount of debris changed and all groups, except group one, recorded a lower level of debris at the recalibration session than at the calibration session. Although debris is a less permanent condition than the other conditions examined, it seems unlikely that this change in measurement could be totally explained by a change in the mouths examined.

Thus, as was found in similar exercises on the previous dental surveys, the measurement of missing and filled teeth proved to be the most reliable.

Table B.1 Calibration and recalibration results for the measurement of different tooth conditions

	Group 1	Group 2	Group 3	Group 4	Group 5	Group 6	Group 7	Group 8
Number of dentists	8	8	8	8	8	8	8	8
Number of subjects	7	7	7	6	7	7	7	8
Missing teeth								
Calibration								
Mean†	46.9	59.6	45.5	39.9	60.3	62.7	53.3	63.9
Standard deviation	0.3	1.4	0.8	0.3	0.7	0.9	0.5	0.4
Coeff of variation*	0.01	0.02	0.02	0.01	0.01	0.01	0.01	0.01
Recalibration								
Mean†	48.1	60.9	45.3	38.5	59.7	64.4	53.4	64
Standard deviation	0.3	0.6	0.5	0.5	0.5	0.7	0.5	—
Coeff of variation*	0.01	0.01	0.01	0.01	0.01	0.01	0.01	—
Filled (otherwise sound) teeth								
Calibration								
Mean†	75.7	95.1	62.9	71.5	66.0	78.9	78.4	90.4
Standard deviation	1.4	2.6	4.6	2.1	2.6	2.5	5.6	3.5
Coeff of variation*	0.02	0.03	0.07	0.03	0.04	0.03	0.07	0.04
Recalibration								
Mean†	74.0	94.9	66.4	74.0	66.5	81.4	81.7	95.1
Standard deviation	3.3	1.6	2.1	2.6	1.8	1.1	3.6	4.1
Coeff of variation*	0.05	0.02	0.03	0.04	0.03	0.01	0.04	0.04
Decayed and filled teeth								
Calibration								
Mean†	4.9	2.8	5.9	4.9	3.0	4.1	5.9	6.9
Standard deviation	2.6	2.5	4.0	2.6	2.3	2.5	5.4	3.6
Coeff of variation*	0.53	0.91	0.68	0.54	0.78	0.61	0.92	0.53
Recalibration								
Mean†	4.9	2.0	3.0	3.5	2.0	2.4	3.3	5.9
Standard deviation	1.8	2.6	1.9	3.2	2.3	0.9	2.6	3.8
Coeff of variation*	0.37	1.28	0.62	0.90	1.16	0.39	0.78	0.65
Decayed, not previously treated teeth								
Calibration								
Mean†	7.6	0.1	6.8	5.5	1.2	2.5	5.4	9.3
Standard deviation	3.9	0.3	1.6	2.6	0.5	1.3	1.4	2.1
Coeff of variation*	0.51	2.83	0.23	0.47	0.37	0.52	0.26	0.23
Recalibration								
Mean†	6.4	0.3	6.9	3.9	1.5	1.2	4.7	8.1
Standard deviation	2.6	0.5	2.4	2.4	0.5	1.0	2.6	3.0
Coeff of variation*	0.41	1.85	0.34	0.62	0.36	0.83	0.54	0.37
All decayed teeth								
Calibration								
Mean†	12.5	2.9	12.6	10.4	4.3	6.6	11.3	16.1
Standard deviation	5.9	2.6	5.3	4.6	2.4	3.1	6.1	5.4
Coeff of variation*	0.47	0.90	0.42	0.44	0.56	0.46	0.54	0.33
Recalibration								
Mean†	11.3	2.2	9.9	7.4	3.5	3.6	8.0	14.0
Standard deviation	3.5	2.4	3.8	4.1	2.1	1.2	4.0	6.4
Coeff of variation*	0.31	1.08	0.39	0.56	0.61	0.33	0.50	0.46

† Mean per dentist

* Coefficient of variation $= \dfrac{Standard\ deviation}{Mean}$

Table B.2 Calibration and recalibration results for the measurement of tooth position

	Group 1	Group 2	Group 3	Group 4	Group 5	Group 6	Group 7	Group 8
Number of dentists	8	8	8	8	8	8	7	7
Number of subjects	7	7	7	6	7	7	7	8
Number of 'spaces'								
Calibration								
Mean†	24.1	9.0	16.7	9.6	13.4	19.0	20.4	13.1
Standard deviation	1.0	2.2	1.9	1.8	1.1	0.8	4.1	2.0
Coeff of variation*	0.04	0.24	0.11	0.19	0.08	0.04	0.20	0.15
Recalibration								
Mean†	26.5	10.9	16.5	10.7	13.3	20.5	20.6	14.4
Standard deviation	1.9	2.9	2.6	2.7	1.2	0.9	4.2	1.5
Coeff of variation*	0.07	0.26	0.15	0.25	0.09	0.05	0.20	0.10
Number of 'no—spaces'								
Calibration								
Mean†	22.7	22.9	23.9	24.1	31.9	23.2	26.9	39.0
Standard deviation	1.2	3.8	2.7	1.5	1.0	1.3	4.3	2.1
Coeff of variation*	0.05	0.17	0.11	0.06	0.03	0.06	0.16	0.05
Recalibration								
Mean†	21.6	22.1	23.1	21.7	31.5	22.7	27.0	37.4
Standard deviation	1.8	3.6	2.2	2.8	1.4	1.5	4.7	1.7
Coeff of variation*	0.08	0.16	0.10	0.13	0.04	0.07	0.17	0.05
Number of segments with crowding								
Calibration								
Mean†	10.5	8.9	8.4	9.0	9.9	7.1	6.6	10.3
Standard deviation	2.2	2.7	2.4	2.5	4.6	2.5	1.9	1.7
Coeff of variation*	0.21	0.30	0.29	0.28	0.47	0.35	0.29	0.17
Recalibration								
Mean†	12.2	7.9	8.0	8.1	9.6	7.5	7.0	10.7
Standard deviation	1.9	2.7	2.5	2.5	7.1	3.0	2.9	3.2
Coeff of variation*	0.16	0.34	0.31	0.31	0.74	0.40	0.42	0.30

† Mean per dentist
* Coefficient of variation $= \dfrac{Standard\ deviation}{Mean}$

Table B.3 Calibration and recalibration results for the measurement of different gum conditions

	Group 1	Group 2	Group 3	Group 4	Group 5	Group 6	Group 7	Group 8
Number of dentists	8	8	8	8	8	8	7	7
Number of subjects	7	7	7	6	7	7	7	8
Debris◊								
Calibration								
Mean†	5.3	8.5	21.5	19.5	7.0	11.3	14.0	19.6
Standard deviation	3.9	4.1	8.5	5.3	6.3	5.3	5.7	6.7
Coeff of variation*	0.74	0.48	0.39	0.27	0.9	0.47	0.41	0.34
Recalibration								
Mean†	6.1	5.0	16.0	17.0	4.1	8.7	11.3	17.4
Standard deviation	5.7	3.3	5.6	5.2	4.6	4.3	10.2	8.0
Coeff of variation*	0.93	0.65	0.35	0.31	1.11	0.49	0.91	0.46
Calculus◊								
Calibration								
Mean†	10.4	6.5	12.5	9.4	12.1	9.0	14.9	10.0
Standard deviation	3.6	2.3	3.9	2.9	4.5	3.4	5.9	3.7
Coeff of variation*	0.35	0.36	0.31	0.31	0.37	0.38	0.40	0.37
Recalibration								
Mean†	8.5	6.9	11.9	9.0	8.3	6.1	12.7	8.0
Standard deviation	3.3	3.1	4.5	4.4	2.7	3.8	3.5	2.5
Coeff of variation*	0.38	0.46	0.38	0.49	0.32	0.62	0.27	0.31
Gingivitis◊								
Calibration								
Mean†	18.8	14.0	22.9	27.1	16.4	13.4	22.9	22.1
Standard deviation	10.9	6.4	5.6	4.7	7.6	5.1	4.6	6.1
Coeff of variation*	0.58	0.46	0.24	0.17	0.47	0.38	0.20	0.28
Recalibration								
Mean†	17.9	15.8	22.1	23.6	12.4	10.6	17.0	21.5
Standard deviation	11.8	5.4	5.7	6.2	7.6	6.3	9.3	8.2
Coeff of variation*	0.66	0.35	0.26	0.26	0.61	0.60	0.55	0.38
Perio◊								
Calibration								
Mean†	2.7	2.9	6.6	0.9	1.3	1.9	5.7	2.3
Standard deviation	2.5	2.0	2.6	1.0	2.1	0.6	3.0	2.2
Coeff of variation*	0.93	0.71	0.39	1.13	1.64	0.34	0.53	0.97
Recalibration								
Mean†	3.5	2.9	5.5	2.0	1.5	1.7	3.4	2.9
Standard deviation	2.6	3.0	3.0	2.0	2.1	1.0	2.0	1.8
Coeff of variation*	0.73	1.06	0.54	1.0	1.4	0.59	0.58	0.62

† Mean per dentist
* Coefficient of variation $= \dfrac{Standard\ deviation}{Mean}$

◊ Number of segments with.....

66

Notes on the oral examination

The criteria for the examination were chosen to ensure that there could be as much comparison as possible with the 1968 study and so that where ever possible the results in this study could be complementary to those obtained in the study of Children's Dental Health in England and Wales 1973. These notes highlight the differences between this and the previous studies.

Training of the examiners
The pattern of training for the dental examiner followed that established for the children's study. It lasted for five working days which was twice the time available in 1968. Each examiner completed about 40 examinations during the training periods for the 1973 and 1978 studies considerably more than in 1968.

Both the training courses in 1973 and 1978 were residential, but in 1978 they were in one place allowing more time to be devoted to the tuition; the major difference between the 1973 and the 1978 training courses was that the system of tutors was introduced. This allowed the time to be utilised effectively and ensure that everyone was thoroughly conversant with the criteria and procedures.

A further difference was in the persons recruited to carry out the examinations. In 1968 dental epidemiology was only undertaken by a few academics, so the majority of the examiners involved had little experience of the techniques and principles involved. Since that time the importance of the discipline has received wide recognition and it now forms a major part of postgraduate courses. In 1978 almost all the examiners involved had experience of such courses and many had undertaken epidemiological projects of their own.

Missing teeth
When examining adults it is very difficult to determine the reason for the loss of teeth which are not present in the mouth. For this reason any tooth which was absent was classified as missing in both the 1968 and 1978 studies. When children are examined the reason for loss is much easier to determine and in the 1973 study the reason for their loss was categorised. Care must therefore be taken when comparing the results of the older children from the 1973 study with the younger adults of this study to ensure that comparisons are not made between teeth missing due to extraction because they were carious in the former and missing due to any reason in the latter.

Dental caries
The criteria for recording the state of the surfaces of each tooth was the same for all three studies.

Periodontal status
One aspect of dental epidemiological work where the experts fail to agree on suitable criteria is in assessing the status of the gums. The visual assessment of changes of shape or colour is inevitably very subjective. Thus the way in which an individual makes their assessment must be affected by their experience of the disease process and the way in which this part of the training programme is presented.

These problems make everyone dissatisfied with existing indices and therefore there is a constant search for something better. For this reason a different set of criteria were used for the children's study than were used in 1968. The differences were both in the indices themselves and the sites at which they were recorded. As many envisaged the problem was not solved and the difficulties remained. As no clear index had emerged at the start of this study a compromise was chosen in the interests of comparability. The sites of examination were chosen to coincide with those used in the children's study and the indices were modified, hopefully to minimize the subjectivity. In addition, expert periodontal advice was sought when the changes were made, and this expert was responsible for this part of the training course.

In addition to these changes it is generally accepted that over the past ten years there has been an increased awareness amongst the dental professions of the subtle visual changes which take place as periodontal disease becomes established.

Orthodontic assessment
Some of the indices used in the children's study for assessing aspects of occlusion had indicated that there was a large need for orthodontic treatment in the older children. These indices were retained in this study to enable the problem to be investigated into adult life.

Dentures
In this study the examination of dentures was restricted to partial dentures. The criteria were the same as those used in 1968 with the omission of those criteria applicable to full dentures. Some new criteria were included which gave information about the design of partial dentures.

The conduct of the examination and criteria for the assessments

The Criteria should be studied in conjunction with the examination form. Name, Date of Birth, Sex, Serial Number and dental status will be completed by the Interviewer before entering the house.

IF THE PATIENT HAS DENTURES THEY WILL BE ASKED TO WEAR THEM FOR THIS PART OF THE EXAMINATION.

1 .   EXISTENCE OF THE TEETH

Permanent teeth will be examined in the following order:

Upper left — upper right — lower right — lower left

Every tooth shown on the chart should be given one of the following codes (ie code all 32 teeth):

P — Present

M — Missing

U — Broken down tooth and definite pulp involvement

C — Crown or temporary crown

Notes:

1. **Codes P and M.** The use of these codes, where the true designation of a tooth may be in doubt, needs some clarification.

The following suggestions may help:

a. Estimate gap sizes, allowing for drifting.

b. Look behind the last standing tooth. Could there have been another tooth there?

c. Look at the tissue in spaces. Is it heaped up, indicating a considerable closure of this space already?

d. Examine the form of the tooth; eg in the upper jaw, third molars are smaller and have a less well-defined cusp pattern.

e. Look at the other quadrants.

f. Ask the patient about loss of teeth.

g. If there is doubt about the identification of the last standing tooth then score the tooth as the second molar, not as the third.

h. If there is a decidious tooth present in the arch then its successor will be scored as M.

2. **Code C.** This is FULL crown. Three-quarter crowns are coded as fillings. In this case use code P.

REPLACEMENT OF MISSING TEETH (Gaps)

Every tooth which has been classified as M in the section above, will be additionally coded into one of the following categories:

D — The tooth has been replaced by a denture or prosthesis which can be removed from the mouth.

B — The tooth has been replaced by a bridge or prosthesis which cannot be removed from the mouth.

N — No space.

S — Space.

Note:

Category N will be used when the remaining space is equal or less than $\frac{1}{2}$ the width of the missing tooth, and for all missing third molars.

AT THIS POINT IN THE EXAMINATION THE PATIENT WILL BE ASKED TO REMOVE THEIR DENTURES.

2 .   DENTURE BEARING AREAS (DBA)

When the patient has removed the denture, the denture-bearing areas will be examined. The examiner will assess whether, in his opinion, the denture itself is having a destructive effect on these tissues. Only those conditions related to the wearing of partial dentures will be assessed eg gum stripping, tilting of teeth and caries on teeth adjacent to the denture. Conditions common to full or partial dentures will not be recorded eg traumatic ulcers, denture stomatitis. The findings will be recorded separately for each denture as follows:

affecting = 1

not affecting = 2

Note:

In the situation where a flabby ridge exists beneath a full upper or lower denture opposed by either natural teeth or a partial denture, this is recorded in this section as 'affecting'.

IF IN DOUBT, SCORE LOW

3 . SURFACES

The teeth which are present will be re-examined in the order given before. Each will be re-identified (to ensure correct recodes) and each surface coded in the order, mesial, occlusal, distal, lingual and buccal. The surfaces are recorded in the following categories:

O — The surface is sound. None of the criteria under X are applicable, and the surface is not filled.

A — The surface is restored with amalgam

G — The surface is restored with gold

S — The surface is restored with a synthetic filling material

X — The surface has decay present, a temporary dressing, or a missing restoration. The surface is regarded as decayed if, in the opinion of the examiner, after visual examination, there is a carious cavity. If doubt exists it will be investigated with the probe supplied and unless the point enters the lesion the surface will be recorded as sound. (O)

Notes:

a. Where a surface has been restored with more than one type of filling material only code the material which occupies the largest area.

b. The code for the filling material, (chosen as in a. if necessary) may be multicoded with X.

c. Chipped or cracked fillings which need replacement are multicoded with the symbol for the major restorative material together with X.

d. Where a filling from one surface encroaches on another, eg an occlusal filling with buccal or lingual extensions, then the filling is charted as being present on all surfaces on to which it extends.

e. New caries at the junction of a filling and the tooth is charted as code X if the criteria for code X are fulfilled. This is multicoded as filling and caries.

f. With rotated teeth identify the anatomical surfaces of the tooth when coding, and not those related to its new position.

g. Do not transilluminate the molar and premolar teeth.

IF IN DOUBT, SCORE LOW

4 . PERIODONTAL STATUS (Gums)

Method of assessment

In applying the scoring methods for soft deposits, calculus, gingivitis and periodontal involvement the mouth is divided into six segments, three upper and three lower, as follows: anterior, from distal surface of canine to distal surface of canine, and left and right posterior from first premolar to the last tooth in the arch, including the interdental papilla distal to the canine. Each assessment should be made independently; soft deposits should all be noted before calculus is recorded, and all recordings of calculus should be made before those of gingivitis or periodontal involvement. The presence or absence of each of these four conditions will be recorded for the upper left posterior segment, then for the upper anterior segment, and finally for the upper right posterior segment. The opposite sequence will be followed for the lower jaw; ie the lower right segment, lower anterior segment and finally the lower left segment.

The lingual and vestibular aspect of each segment should be inspected for each assessment. All assessments in a particular segment should cease when a condition is detected on any aspect of any tooth in that segment.

Criteria for assessment and coding

A. Soft Deposits

The only instrument to be used is a mouth mirror. If soft deposits are clearly visible to the unaided eye at the gingival margin of one or more teeth within a segment, score '1' for that segment. No attempt should be made to dry the teeth to make soft deposits more readily apparent. If no soft deposit is detected visually within a segment, score '0' for that segment.

B. Calculus (Supragingival)

Score '1' for a segment when calculus is obviously present in contact with the gingival margin of one or more teeth in the segment. Any obvious deposit suspected of being calculus when assessed by direct inspection or with the aid of a mouth mirror, should be tested with a periodontal probe to confirm that it is in fact calcified, and a score of '1' is then recorded. If the deposit is not calcified score '0'.

C. Gingivitis

The state of the gums will be coded according to one of the following criteria:

0 —   The gums appear healthy; pale pink and firm with no evidence of inflammation. (No treatment is indicated).

1 —   Moderate gingivitis: The gingival margin is redder and may be slightly oedematous. There is no tendency to bleed. (In this case the gingivitis should respond to plaque control alone).

2 —   Intense gingivitis: The gingivae are markedly red and oedematous. They bleed on digital pressure. (Only if doubt exists in this category should an attempt be made to elicit bleeding) (Plaque control alone may not be sufficient to resolve the condition).

Certain gingival conditions exist which, although scoring '0' or '1' on the gingivitis assessment, require more than plaque control alone to resolve the condition. These should be given the appropriate gingival score plus an asterisk and details recorded in Comments (eg Gingival hyperplasia). This should be recorded for each segment involved.

Mucosal trauma, due to incisors biting on the palatal gingiva or labial gingiva should be marked as an asterisk and recorded in Comments.

D. Periodontitis

A segment will be examined for one of or both the following conditions:

1. Gingivitis category 2, as defined above
2. Marked changes in gingival contour

If either or both the above conditions exist, periodontitis is suspected in that segment. In this case proceed as follows:

1. Test for definite tooth mobility. If mobility is found **Score 1**, otherwise proceed to
2. The periodontal probe is used on all tooth surfaces which fulfill the criteria for **PERIODONTITIS** in D to detect pockets greater in depth than 3 mm beyond the amelo-cemental junction. If such a pocket is found then **Score 1** for that segment.

Note:

In the case of doubt in any of the above conditions then the lower category should be recorded.

5 . CROWDING

Assessment of crowding is to be made on teeth erupted into the oral cavity at that time and no account taken of missing teeth and/or potential crowding. Each segment is to be recorded separately, the middle segments to include incisors and canines, and the right and left segments to include premolars and molars. Record in the following categories:

0 —   No crowding, the standing teeth fit into that segment of the dental arch without overlapping or irregularity.

1 —   There is a shortage of space or overlap or irregularity in that segment of not more than one premolar width (left and right segments), or one lower lateral incisor width (lower middle segment), or one upper lateral incisor width (upper middle segment).

2 — There is a shortage of space or overlap or irregularity in that segment to a greater extent than in the previous category (1).

IF IN DOUBT, SCORE LOW

OCCLUSAL ASSESSMENT

The assessment of overbite and overjet should be made only when there is sufficient posterior support for the patient to maintain a consistent occlusion and where natural incisor teeth are present. The assessment is to be made therefore with the denture out, the teeth in centric occlusion, and the Frankfort plane horizontal.

6 . OVERJET

This is the horizontal distance in mms between the labial surfaces of the upper and lower central incisors. The general incisor relationship should first be assessed ie if the majority are proclined then score as positive, if retroclined, score as negative, and if edge-to-edge as zero. Then a measurement should be made with the gauge supplied on the central incisors with the greatest displacement in the same direction as the general displacement. When no assessment is possible, the recorder will strike through this part of the form. If the assessment falls between marks on the gauge, record the lower mark.

7 . OVERBITE

This is the amount by which the upper incisors overlap the lower incisors in the vertical dimension. The overbite should be assessed at the level of the centre of the incisal edge of the upper left central incisor. If this tooth is missing or instanding, assess on the right upper central incisor. If no assessment is possible, the recorder will strike through this part of the form. Assess and record the proportion of the crowns of the lower incisor overlapped by the upper incisor in the following categories:

1 — The upper incisor does not overlap the lower incisor.

2 — The upper incisor overlaps the lower incisor by not more than one-third of the clinical crown of the lower incisor.

3 — The upper incisor overlaps the lower incisor by more than one-third of the clinical crown of the lower incisor.

IF IN DOUBT, SCORE LOW

8 . TRAPPED LOWER LIP

If the lower lip rests passively behind the natural upper incisors record as:

1 — trapped

0 — not trapped

IF IN DOUBT, SCORE LOW

9 . DENTURES

The dentures, including those full dentures opposed by natural teeth or a partial denture will then be examined and the following recorded for each:

(i) **Dentures**

Partial — 1

Full — 2

(ii) **Denture Material**

Metal — Those dentures where the major component of the fitting surface is metal not including those whose only metal component is clasps.

Plastic — Dentures whose major component is plastic.

(iii) **Denture Type**

Tooth borne — Dentures with bounded saddles and rests.

Tissue borne — Dentures without rests.

Both — Dentures with rests and free-end saddles.

(iv) **Denture State**

Complete

Broken — Where the denture is in need of repair eg fractured, tooth missing or self-mended.

(v) **Denture Hygiene**

If, in the dentist's opinion, there is no debris on the denture ie no plaque, calculus and staining record as:

1 —   Satisfactory (Satis)

If there is debris record as:

2 —   Not satisfactory (Not)

If the denture is clean apart from staining or recent food debris, score 1.

(vi) **Replacement**

If, in the dentist's opinion, the denture needs to be replaced score as:

1 —   Replacement required

0 —   No replacement required

(vii) **Number of Margins**

This is the number of lingual or palatal margins covered by the denture. When half a margin is covered, count as 1. If it is not possible accurately to count the number of collets on the denture, then it should be reinserted and a check made in the mouth, against the teeth.

IF IN DOUBT, SCORE LOW

10.   ASTERISKS (DENTISTS' COMMENTS)

The dentist will be asked if he wishes to make any comments. If so, they will be recorded on the back of the form by the dentist. Comments should be restricted to those conditions requiring the intervention of a dentist, which have not already been recorded on the front of the form. (The check list should be used in order to confine the range of comments to those relevant ie expressing a treatment need.)

CHECK LIST

Impacted wisdom teeth and/or pericoronitis

Rotated incisor teeth

Supernumerary teeth

Hypodontia

Development anomalies of enamel/dentine

Clefts of lip and/or palate

Gingival hyperplasia

Abscesses

Diseases of oral mucous membrane

Mucosal trauma

Acknowledgements

We would like to thank the University of Birmingham for allowing us to participate in the study and the Birmingham Dental School and Hospital for the use of facilities. We are grateful to the technical and secretarial staff of the Dental School who assisted in the preparation of teaching material for the training courses, participated in the pre-pilot study and ably helped with the administrative arrangements. To those members of staff who allowed us to examine a few of their patients during the pre-pilot study and to those who lent us slides and models for teaching purposes, and in particular, Professor R M Basker for his help in devising and interpreting the criteria in relation to the section dealing with Prosthetics, we extend our thanks.

We are indebted to Proctor and Gamble for the use of their research establishment during the training programme in particular, to Mr D Delahunt, Director, Product Development and Mr H Trainer, Manager, Toilet Goods Product Development for making this possible. Also the many members of their staff who so willingly agreed to act as subjects for the dental examinations, not only for the main training programme but also for the pilot study and the recalibration exercise. Without their co-operation, such a task would have been impossible. We are specially grateful to Mr L Ness, Professional and Regulatory Service Specialist whose untiring and ceaseless activity coupled with impeccable organisation guaranteed us a constant supply of subjects to an examination environment as near ideal as was humanly possible.

We would have been severely hampered in our training of so many examiners if it had not been for the invaluable assistance of the four area dental officers, Mr R Bettles, Mr J Onions, Mr J Palmer and Mr F I H Whitehead, all of whom participated in the pilot study. We extend our thanks to them for their unfailing help throughout.

Our thanks are due also to Ms G Bradnock whose organisational skills ensured the smooth running of each stage of the entire training programme, from the pre-pilot study to the recalibration exercise.

We extend our thanks to Colgate-Palmolive and those of their employees who agreed to undergo the reproducibility exercise that Dr M Downer and Ms G Bradnock carried out with the two lighting systems.

Finally, we wish to express our gratitude to all those dentists who so willingly underwent a most rigorous training programme and without whose full co-operation the study would not have been possible. They are listed in Annex 2.

Annex 1 The dental examination kit.

4 plane mouth mirrors
4 dental explorers, blunted to 0.7mm
1 orthodontic measure
1 chip syringe
4 flexible examination lights

2 beakers, with lids
1 plastic bag
1 sponge
2 towels
1 portable case

Annex 2 The dentists taking part

Mr A Bewick
Mr R Blankenstein
Mrs W Boyles
Mrs V Burke
Mrs M Chalmers
Mr G Crawford
Mr R L Davies
Mr G J Derbyshire
Mr J Docherty
Mr J E Donald
Dr M C Downer
Mr M M M F D'Souza
Mr C K Fenton-Evans
Mr M R Fishwick
Mr C J Frodsham
Mr W H Garland

Mr R M Gray
Mr P Gore
Mr P A Hancock
Mr S A Hancocks
Mr J E Hartley
Mr F C Hodgson
Mr J Horn
Mr M E Jenkins
Mr A M Jenner
Miss P A King
Mr A Mckendrick
Mrs G P Mckendrick
Mr K S McPhail
Mr R Maxwell
Miss S M Miller
Mr K J Moss

Miss R C Nesbitt
Mr J Newman
Mr J E F Nixon
Mr M Parkhouse-Evans
Mr W Quirke
Mr J Rhodes
Mr R Rippon
Mrs K H Rothwell
Mr P Rowley
Miss R A Russell
Miss E J Salisch
Miss S Sandham
Mr W Smith
Mr D K Stables
Mr C J D Sykes
Mr J F G Thomas

Mr N Thomas
Mr G Thompson
Mr D Traini
Mr G H Tucker
Miss D Wieczorek
Mr J W Langford
Mr T S Longworth
Mr H Lunn
Mr R H Willets
Mr D Williams
Mr M Williams
Mrs S Williams
Mrs P D Wilson
Mr K Woods
Mr N Wylie

Appendix C   A comparison of dental examinations using the different illumination systems employed in the 1968 and 1978 Surveys of Adult Dental Health.

Martin C. Downer, PhD, LDS, DDPH,

University of Manchester Dental Health Unit.

A study was conducted to test the null hypothesis that there was no systematic error between dental examinations performed with a battery operated head lamp, used in the 1968 survey of adult dental health, and the battery operated intraoral 'Flexible Examination Light'* used in the 1978 survey.

Material and Method

Two series of examinations were conducted two weeks apart on a volunteer group of factory employees. The same subjects were examined on both occasions, once using the headlamp and once using the intraoral light. Thirty subjects were originally scheduled for examination but because of absence from work the number who eventually received both examinations was 19. The results are confined to these. The subjects were all dentate males or females over sixteen years of age. They included both office and technical staff and workers from the shop floor. Patients who attended the industrial dental practice located in the factory were excluded.

To allow for systematic error from a possible shift in the examiner's diagnostic standards between the first and second series of examinations, the sequence in which the lights were used was varied. The order of use was decided with a table of random numbers. Thus on the first occasion nine subjects were examined with the intraoral light and ten with the headlamp, while on the second occasion subjects were examined with the alternative light source.

The method of examination was that described in Appendix B of this report. The occlusal assessment and examination of dentures were excluded because these parts of the examination were considered unlikely to be affected by the type of illumination used.

The only departure from strict adherence to the field method was that the examinations were conducted in a dental surgery with the subjects reclining in the dental chair and the examiner seated. Natural and artificial background light supplemented the main source of intraoral illumination as in the field examinations. Apart from the chair and operating stool, no other facilities available in the surgery were used. The examiner had undergone a course of training and calibration attended by survey examiners the week preceding the study. He was assisted by an experienced recording scribe.

* Hoyt Laboratories Division of Colgate Palmolive Limited.

Measurements of decayed tooth surfaces, filled and carious surfaces, soft organic material, supragingival calculus, gingivitis, and segments with periodontal pockets were collected and analysed. Unadjusted mean scores from the two series of examinations are reported. For each factor, the data were subjected to an incomplete three-way analysis of variance to examine the effects both of type of light and the sequence in which the lights were used. In addition correlation coefficients were calculated between the scores obtained with each type of light. All computations were carried out by hand.

Results

The table of results presents the mean whole mouth scores obtained with the two different sources of illumination for each of the seven conditions considered, together with the mean differences between scores. The values of the coefficients of correlation (Pearson's r) between the two series of 19 measurements are given and also the F values for the differences between lights, between the sequences of their use and for interaction between light sequence.

There was no statistically significant difference between scores obtained with the two illumination systems for any of the conditions included, and in no instance did the mean difference exceed one tooth surface or one affected segment of the mouth.

In all comparisons, with the exception of those for supragingival calculus and gingivitis, higher scores were obtained with the intraoral light than the headlamp. In percentage terms, for example, some 30 per cent more unrestored surfaces were diagnosed as carious with the intraoral light. However, in several instances, whether the measurement was obtained on the first or the second occasion of examination proved more important than the type of light used. Quoting again the example of decay without restoration, 65 per cent more surfaces were scored carious at the second examination than at the first, although this represented a mean difference of only 0.68 of a surface. It is evident that the systematic difference between the scores obtained on each occasion often exceeded the systematic difference arising from the lights. This is reflected, in several of the comparisons, in the higher F values for the sequence in which the lights were used and the light and sequence interaction than the F values for differences between the lights. Apart from decayed surfaces, this situation was apparent for filled and carious surfaces, gingivitis, and for segments with soft organic deposits. The table shows that the interaction of the type of light and the sequence of use was statistically significant ($P<0.05$) for this last factor.

The coefficients of correlation ranged from r = 1.00, representing almost perfect correlation for the number of surfaces scored with each type of light as filled and sound, down to r = 0.23 for segments with periodontal pockets. The correlation coefficients for conditions associated with the periodontium were all lower than those for restored surfaces and decayed surfaces.

Discussion and Conclusions

From the results of this study, the null hypothesis of no systematic differences between measurements of dental conditions obtained with the intraoral light and the headlamp cannot be rejected. However, although with the limited number of subjects available in this study no statistically significant differences could be detected between the two lights, such differences as did occur might be considered important if magnified in a large sample. An increase in the recorded level of unrestored surfaces with caries of 30 per cent for example resulting from use of the new illumination system, might render comparisons of the findings of the 1968 and 1978 surveys of adult dental health questionable, although such a difference amounts to only slightly over one third of a tooth surface.

On the other hand, a systematic shift in the diagnostic standards of the examiner was found to be generally greater than the bias arising from the differences in illumination. Field examinations are likely to be no less prone to this type of error than those conducted in an experimental situation.

It may be concluded that although higher scores were obtained for most dental conditions with the intraoral light than the headlamp, the mean differences were in general small. Bias arising from the use of the improved illumination system is likely to be less than that arising from fluctuations in diagnostic levels and almost certainly less than systematic differences occurring between a number of examiners in a field survey.

Acknowledgements

Thanks are due to Colgate Palmolive Limited for permitting and facilitating this study, particularly Mr. Graham Davies for his help with the organisation, and the employees who took part in the examinations. The assistance of Miss Gillian Bradnock of the University of Birmingham is also gratefully acknowledged.

Table C.1 Results

	Intraoral light (mean)	Headlamp (mean)	Difference (mean)	Pearson's r	F value between lights	F value between sequences of use	F value for light and sequence interaction
Carious surfaces	1.58	1.21	+0.37	0.90	0.10	2.72	3.25
Filled and carious	0.63	0.53	+0.10	0.91	0.40	1.33	1.52
Filled and sound	21.95	21.16	+0.79	1.00	1.35	0.01	0.00
Segments with soft organic deposits	1.47	1.42	+0.05	0.83	0.06	1.01	6.65*
Segments with supragingival calculus	0.58	0.68	—0.10	0.69	0.40	0.01	1.52
Segments with gingivitis	2.37	2.58	—0.21	0.47	0.13	0.28	2.60
Segments with periodontal pockets	1.00	0.42	+0.58	0.23	2.04	1.12	0.53

* $P < 0.05$

Appendix D: The questionnaires

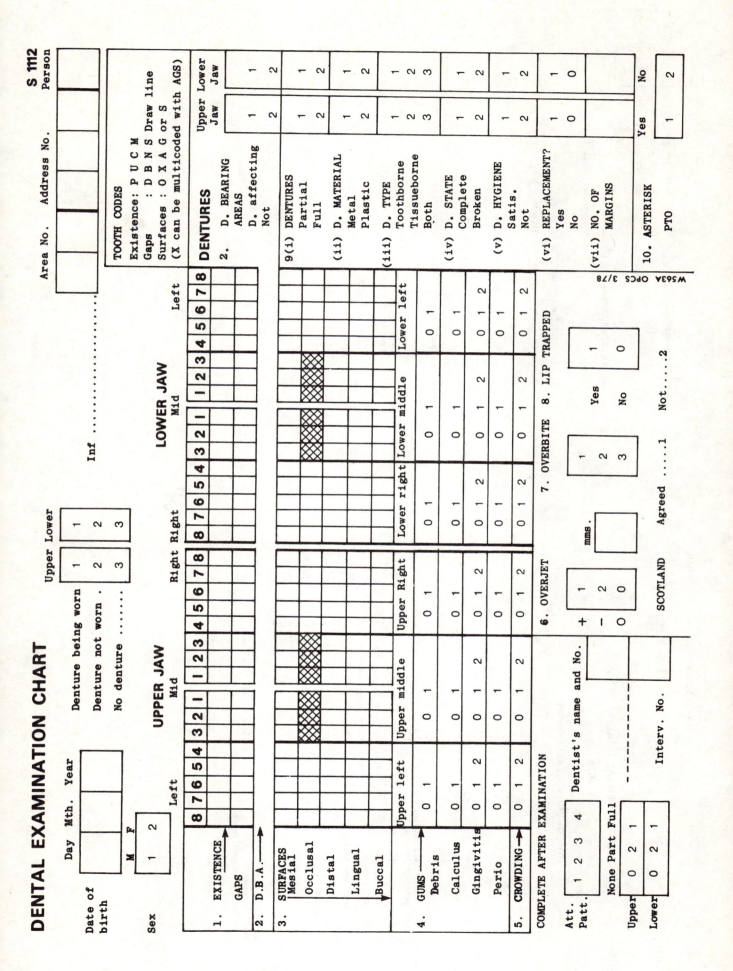

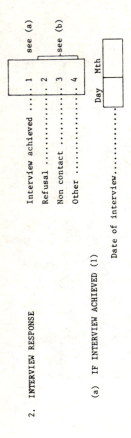

Area No.   Address No.   Person

S1112

ADULT DENTAL HEALTH
UK 1978

Introductory questionnaire

Interviewer's name..........   Inf.............

Interviewer's no...........

(We are interested in all people, those with all natural teeth, those with some false teeth and those with all false teeth)

1 Could you tell me have you still got some of your natural teeth or have you lost them all?

Still has some natural teeth..	4	ask (a)
Lost them all..............	3	go to GREEN Q'RE

IF HAS SOME NATURAL TEETH (4)

(a) Have you ever had any dentures, that is false teeth on a plate?

Has had dentures.....	4	ask (b)
Never had dentures...	1	go to YELLOW Q'RE

IF HAS HAD DENTURES (4)

(b) Can I just check, have you ever had both a full upper and a full lower plate?

Both full upper and full lower.	3	go to GREEN Q'RE
Has not.............	2	go to PINK Q'RE

INTERVIEWER SEE OVER PAGE

---

2. INTERVIEW RESPONSE

Interview achieved	1 see (a)
Refusal	2 see (b)
Non contact	3
Other	4

Date of interview...........   Day Mth

(a) IF INTERVIEW ACHIEVED (1)

(b) IF INTERVIEW NOT ACHIEVED (2, 3 or 4)

Please Give Best Estimate of Informant's Age, Sex and Dental Status

Age				Sex			Dental Status		
16-34	35-54	55+	DK	M	F	DK	Some natural teeth	No natural teeth	DK
1	2	3	4	1	2	3	1	2	3

3. DENTAL EXAMINATION RESPONSE

Informant has no natural teeth	1	see (a)
Informant has some natural teeth — Examination achieved	2	
Refusal at end of interview	3	
Refusal later	4	
Non contact for examination	5	
Other	6	

(a) IF EXAMINATION ACHIEVED (2)

Date of dental examination.....   Day Mth

Time of day for dental examination

Before 2 o'clock..............	1
2 o'clock but before 5 o'clock....	2
5 o'clock or later............	3

W560 OPCS 3/78

S1112

Area No.	Address No.				Person

ADULT DENTAL HEALTH

UK 1978

Interview questionnaire 1

People with natural teeth only

Interviewer's Name ....   Inf. ....

Interviewer's No. ....

I'd like to start by talking about how your teeth are at the moment.

1. Many people suffer from toothache at one time or another. During the last four weeks have you had a toothache at all or not?

Had toothache ...	1
Not	2

2. During the last four weeks have you lost any fillings or have any bits broken off your teeth?

Fillings lost/tooth broken.	1
None	2

3. Do you think any of your teeth are at all loose?

Some loose	1
None	2

4. When you are eating or drinking are there any teeth that you avoid using?

Avoids some ...	1 → ask (a)
Does not	2

   IF AVOIDS SOME (1)
   (a) What is the main reason for you avoiding those teeth?

5. (Can I just check) do you think any of your teeth are decayed at the moment?

Teeth decayed	1
Not	2

1

Dental health is not only to do with teeth but with gums as well

6 Are your gums swollen at all at the moment?

Gums swollen .. 1
Not 2

7 Are your gums inflamed, that is redder than usual, at the moment?

Gums inflamed 1
Not............. 2

8 During the last four weeks have your gums bled at all for example when you brushed your teeth or at any other time?

Gums bled 1
Have not 2

9 Do you have any other sort of trouble with your gums at the moment?

Other trouble 1   ask (a)
Not 2

IF OTHER TROUBLE (1)
(a) What other trouble do you have?

10 If you were to go to the dentist tomorrow do you think you would need any treatment or not?

Need treatment 1   ask (a)
Not 2

IF NEED TREATMENT (1)
(a) What sort of treatment do you think you would need?
PROMPT AS NEC.
CODE ALL THAT APPLY

Fillings 1
Extractions 2
Fillings/extractions but dk which .. 3
Other (SPECIFY) 4

11(a) If you went to the dentist with an aching back tooth would you prefer the dentist to take it out or to fill it?
PROMPT AS NEC. "Supposing it could be filled"

Take it out ... 1
Fill it 2
Other 3
(SPECIFY)

(b) If you went to the dentist with an aching front tooth would you prefer the dentist to take it out or to fill it?
PROMPT AS NEC. "Supposing it could be filled"

Take it out ... 1
Fill it 2
Other 3
(SPECIFY)

2

12 You told me earlier that you've never had any dentures but when people lose some of their own teeth they may need a denture to replace them.

(a) Do you find the thought of having a partial denture to replace some of your natural teeth ....
RUNNING PROMPT

.....very upsetting .. 1
a little upsetting .. 2
or not at all upsetting .. 3

(b) A lot of people eventually have their own teeth out and have full dentures. Do you find the thought of losing all your own teeth and having full dentures ...
RUNNING PROMPT

.....very upsetting .. 1
a little upsetting .. 2
or not at all upsetting .. 3

13 Do you think at sometime you will have to have full dentures or do you think you will always keep some of your natural teeth?

Have full dentures ... 1   ask (a)
Keep natural teeth ... 2
D.K. 3

IF HAVE FULL DENTURES (1)
(a) At what age do you think you'll first need full dentures?
PROMPT AS NECESSARY

70's or more .. 7
60's 6
50's 5
40's 4
30's 3
20's 2

14 Thinking of the people you know around your age about how many of them have full dentures; would you say it was ...
RUNNING PROMPT

All or most of them... 1
Some of them 2
very few or none of them. 3

15 Whether or not teeth are lost is due partly to how healthy they are and different people have different ideas as to what things help to keep teeth healthy. I'd like to talk about some things people have mentioned. Can you tell me how important you consider them for keeping teeth healthy.

HAND OVER CARD A

FOR KEEPING TEETH HEALTHY				
very important	fairly important	not very important	not at all important	D.K.

Would you say that ......

	very important	fairly important	not very important	not at all important	D.K.
(i) Not eating sweets is.....	1	2	3	4	5
(ii) Regular visits to the dentist are	1	2	3	4	5
(iii) Cleaning teeth regularly is	1	2	3	4	5
(iv) Having fluoride in the water is	1	2	3	4	5

3

Now I'd like to talk a little about cleaning your teeth

16(a) How often do you clean your teeth nowadays?

Never	9	go to Q.17
Once a day ...	1
Twice a day .	2
More than twice a day ..	3
..............per............ Other (SPECIFY) ...	4

(b) At what time of day do you clean them?

Before breakfast 1
After breakfast 2
Midday 3
Tea time 4
After evening meal ... 5
Last thing at night ... 6
Other (SPECIFY) 7

IF MORNING AND NO BREAKFAST RING 'AFTER BREAKFAST' (2)

(c) About how long ago did you start using the toothbrush you've got now? Was it ...

less than 3 months 1
3 months, but less than 6 months 2
6 months, but less than a year 3
or a year or more ago? 4
D.K 5
No toothbrush 6

(e) Do you use toothpaste, toothpowder or something else to clean your teeth?

Toothpaste ... 1 — ask (f)
Toothpowder .. 2
Other .... 3 — ask (g)
(SPECIFY)

IF TOOTHPASTE OR TOOTHPOWDER (1 or 2)
(f) thinking of the toothpaste (toothpowder) you use at the moment does it contain fluoride or not?

Contains fluoride . 1 — ask (g)
Does not 2
Don't know 3

(g) (Can I just check) do you ever use anything else to clean your teeth such as dental floss or woodsticks?

Dental floss...... 1
Woodsticks 2
Other (SPECIFY) ... 3

4

Can I talk now about your childhood dental experiences

17 When you were a child how much encouragement were you given to clean your teeth? Were you given ....

a great deal 1
a fair amount 2
not much 3
or no encouragement at all? ... 4

18 When you were a child (that is before you were 16) did you ever go to a dentist?

Went to a dentist ..... 1 — ask(a)
Did not .... 2 — go to Q 19

IF WENT TO A DENTIST (1)
(a) Did you go to the school dentist, to some other dentist or both?

School dentist .... 1 — ask(c)
Other dentist .... 2 — ask(b)
Both 3

IF WENT TO OTHER DENTIST OR BOTH (2)(3)
(b) (Excluding visits to the school dentist) as a child, did you go to the dentist for ...

.... a regular check up ... 1
an occasional check up. 2
or only when you were having trouble with your teeth? ...... 3 — ask(c)
Other (SPECIFY) 4

(c) Thinking now about any treatment you had then. Did you have any teeth filled before you were 16?

Teeth filled 1
Not 2
DK/can't remember 3

(d) Did you have any teeth taken out when you were that age?

Teeth taken out 1
Not 2
DK/can't remember 3

(e) Nowadays children sometimes have a brace fitted or teeth taken out to help straighten their teeth. Did you have any treatment to straighten or improve the appearance of your teeth?

Had treatment ..... 1 — ask(f)
Did not 2
DK/can't remember 3

IF HAD TREATMENT (1)
(f) Did you have a brace fitted, teeth taken out, both of these or some other treatment?

Brace fitted 1
Teeth taken out .. 2
Both 3
Other (SPECIFY) ... 4

5

We've talked a little about childhood and now I'd like to talk about the dental experiences you've had through the whole of your life.
IF TEETH FILLED WHEN CHILD (Q18(c) CODE (1)) RING (1) AND ASK (a-b)

19 Have you ever had any teeth filled?

Teeth filled 1   ask (a-b)
Not 2   Go to Q20

IF TEETH FILLED (1)
(a) Have you ever had an injection in your gum to kill the pain of a filling?

Injection in gum 1   ask(c)
Not 2   see(c)

(b) Have you ever had an injection in your arm to kill the pain of a filling?

Injection in arm 1   ask(c)
Not 2   see(c)

IF HAD INJECTION (a) OR (b) CODE (1)
(c) Do you usually have an injection when you're having a filling done?

Usually 1
Not 2

IF TEETH TAKEN OUT WHEN CHILD (Q18 (d) CODE (1)) RING (1) AND ASK (a-c)

20 Have you ever had any teeth taken out?

Teeth taken out 1   ask (a-c)
Not 2   Go to Q21

IF TEETH TAKEN OUT (1)
(a) Have you ever had gas to have teeth taken out?

Had gas 1
Not 2

(b) Have you ever had an injection in your gum to have teeth taken out?

Injection in gum .. 1
Not 2

(c) Have you ever had an injection in your arm to have teeth taken out?

Injection in arm 1
Not 2

21 Have you ever had an Xray taken of your teeth?

Had Xray 1   ask (a)
Not 2

IF HAD XRAY (1)
(a) Do you usually have an Xray taken of your teeth when you go to the dentist?

Usually has Xray 1
Does not 2

22 The wisdom teeth, which are the very back teeth, often come through later than the other teeth and sometimes don't come through at all. Can you tell me which of your wisdom teeth have, at sometime, come through.
Has the one at the ... come through or not?

	top left	top right	bottom left	bottom right
Come through	1	1	1	1
Not come through ..	2	2	2	2
DK	3	3	3	3
still got it	4	4	4	4
taken out ..	5	5	5	5

IF COME THROUGH (1)
(a) Have you still got the ... wisdom tooth or have you had it out since?   ask (a)

As well as treating people's teeth dentists can give advice to their patients on caring for their teeth and mouths and on preventing disease.

23. Has a dentist or any of his staff ever demonstrated to you the best way to clean your teeth?

Demonstrated 1   ask(a)
Not 2

IF DEMONSTRATED (1)
(a) Who was it who demonstrated teeth cleaning to you? Was it ...

... a dentist 1
a dental nurse or hygienist . 2
RUNNING
PROMPT   or somebody else (SPECIFY) 3

24 Has a dentist or any of his staff ever given you any advice on caring for your gums?

Given advice 1   ask(a-b)
Not 2

IF GIVEN ADVICE (1)
(a) Who was it who give you the advice? Was it ...

a dentist 1
a dental nurse or hygienist . 2
or somebody else (SPECIFY) 3

(b) What advice did he/she give you?

25 Has a dentist or any of his staff ever advised you about eating sweets or other sugary things?

Advised 1   ask(a-b)
Not 2

IF ADVISED (1)
(a) Who was it who gave you the advice? Was it .....

a dentist 1
a dental nurse or hygienist . 2
or somebody else (SPECIFY) 3

(b) What did he/she say?

Another part of dentist's work is to provide treatment to improve the appearance of teeth which are crooked or protruding.

SHOW CARD A

26(a) How important do you think it is that children with crooked or protruding teeth should have them straightened. Do you think it is ..

RUNNING PROMPT

... very important	1	
fairly important ..	2	
not very important	3	
or not at all important?.	4	

(b) How important do you think it is that adults with crooked or protruding teeth should have them straightened. Do you think it is ..

RUNNING PROMPT

..very important	1	
fairly important ..	2	
not very important	3	see (c)
or not at all important?.	4	

IF ONE LESS IMPORTANT THAN OTHER
(c) Why do you think it is less important for '..... to have their teeth straightened?

27 How do you feel about your own teeth are you satisfied or not satisfied with the way they look?

Satisfied	1	go to Q28
Not satisfied .	2	ask (a–b)

IF NOT SATISFIED (2)
(a) What is it about the way your teeth look that you're not satisfied with?

(b) Have you ever talked to a dentist about the appearance of your teeth?

Talked to dentist	1	ask (c)
Not	2	ask (d)

IF TALKED TO DENTIST (1)
(c) What did the dentist say?

IF NOT (2)
(d) Is there any reason why you haven't talked to a dentist about the appearance of your teeth?

8

I'd like to talk now about going to the dentist

28 Have you been to the dentist since the beginning of November(December) that's about six months ago?

Yes	1	ask(a)
No	2	ask(b)

IF YES (1)
(a) (Can I just check) are you in the middle of a course of treatment now or not?

In middle of treatment .	1	go to Q29
Not	2	

IF NO (2)
(b) Have you been to the dentist since last April (May/June),that's about a year ago?

Yes	1	go to Q29
No	2	ask(c)

IF NO (b) CODE (2)
(c) About how long ago was your last visit to the dentist?
PROMPT IF NEC.

More than 1 up to 2 years ago	1	ask(d)
More than 2 up to 3 years ago	2	go to Q29
More than 3 up to 5 years ago	3	
More than that (SPECIFY)	4	
Never	5	go to Q 150

IF Q28(c) CODE (1)
(d) Was this before or after April 1st 1977.

Before April 1st	1
April 1st or after	2

29 The last time you went to the dentist what made you go? Was it because you were having some trouble with your teeth or for a check up or for some other reason?

Trouble with teeth ..	1	ask(a)
Check up	2	
Other (SPECIFY)	3	

IF TROUBLE WITH TEETH (1)
(a) Did you have toothache or did you have some other trouble with your teeth?

Toothache	1
Other ...... (SPECIFY)	2

30 When people go to the dentist for a check up or because they've got trouble with their teeth, they sometimes have to make more than one visit for the dentist to carry out any treatment they might need.
When you last went to the dentist how many visits did you have to make?

One visit	1
Two visits	2
Three visits	3
Four visits	4
Five or more	5

9

31

(Can I just check) during the visit(s) you made to the dentist for that course of treatment did you have any...

INDIVIDUAL PROMPT	Yes	No	DK
... X rays taken	1	2	3
Teeth filled	1	2	3
Teeth taken out	1	2	3
Teeth scaled (scraped, cleaned) and polished ...	1	2	3
Other treatment (SPECIFY) ...	1	2	3

32

Was your treatment under the National Health Service, was it private or was it something else?

National Health Service...	1	ask (b)
Private...........	2	ask (a-b)
N.H.S. and private.......	3	
Community Dental Service..	4	
Armed Forces...........	5	
Other (SPECIFY).........	6	

IF N.H.S. AND PRIVATE (3)

(a) What treatment did you have privately?

IF ANY PRIVATE (2 or 3)

(b) What was the main reason for you having this treatment done privately?

33

How much did the treatment cost you?

Cost (SPECIFY)..	1	ask (a)
Nothing.........	2	ask (b)
DK.............	3	go to Q34

IF PAID FOR TREATMENT (1)

(a) Did the treatment cost more than you expected, about what you expected or less than you expected?

More than expected..	1	go to Q34
About what expected..	2	
Less than expected..	3	
Other (SPECIFY).....	4	

IF NOTHING (2)

(b) Why didn't it cost you anything?

No treatment........	1	go to Q34
Under 21, pregnant or nursing mother.......	2	ask (c)
Other (SPECIFY).......	3	

PROMPT AS NEC.

(c) When you went to the dentist did you expect the treatment would be free?

Yes.....	1
No......	2

34

Thinking about the dental practice you went to for your last treatment, was that the first time you had been to that dentist or group of dentists or had you been there before?

First time	1	ask (c)
Been before ...	2	ask (a-b)

IF BEEN BEFORE (2)

(a) For about how many years have you been going to that dentist or group of dentists?

Less than a year	1
One year less than two ...	2
Two years less than five .	3
Five years or more	4
DK/Can't remember	5

(b) Does the dentist sent you a reminder when it is time to go for your next check up?

Sends reminder	1	Go to Q35
Does not	2	ask (c)

IF DOES NOT SEND REMINDER (2) OR FIRST TIME (1)

(c) When you make an appointment to see the dentist do you usually make it ....

... at the end of your previous treatment	1	go to Q35
some time before the date that you want the appointment	2	ask(d)
or when you want to see the dentist as soon as possible	3	
Other (SPECIFY)	4	go to Q35

IF CODE (2) OR (3)

(d) Last time you wanted to see the dentist about how long did you have to wait for an appointment?

35

How did you come to choose that particular dentist?

Can't remember	9

36. In the last five years have you had any difficulty getting any treatment under the National Health Service?

Had difficulty ... 1   ask (a-b)
Not 2
Not tried 3

IF HAD DIFFICULTY (1)
(a) What treatment couldn't you get?

ALL OF IT/
PART OF IT
IF PART WHAT PART?

(b) What did you do about it?

37. In general do you go to the dentist for ...

.. a regular check up 1   Go to Q38
an occasional check up 2
or only when you're having trouble with your teeth ... 3   ask (a-b)

IF DOES NOT GO FOR A REGULAR CHECK UP (2 or 3)
(a) What is the main reason for you not going for a regular check up?

(b) (You've told me the main reason for you not going for a regular check up) now I'd like to ask about the kinds of circumstances when you would go to the dentist. Would you go to the dentist if you had ....

	YES	NO
Occasional twinges of toothache	1	2
A tooth which felt loose	1	2
Not been to the dentist for a long time	1	2
A swollen face	1	2
Sore gums	1	2
Toothache which kept you awake at night	1	2
A gumboil	1	2
A tooth with a piece broken off	1	2
Gums which bled occasionally	1	2

INDIVIDUAL PROMPT

38. Would you say that nowadays you go to the dentist more often, about the same or less often that you did five year ago?

More often 1   ask (a)
About the same 2
Less often 3   ask (a)

IF MORE OR LESS OFTEN (1 or 3)
(a) What has made you go more (less) often?

12

I'd like to talk generally now about the cost of dental treatment under the National Health Service.

39. When you go to the dentist to have treatment do you normally have some idea of how much it's going to cost you?

Has some idea 1
Does not 2

40. Do you know where you can find out about National Health Service dental charges?

Yes 1   ask (a
No 2

IF YES (1)
(a) Where can you find out?

Dentist 1
G.P.O. 2
Other (SPECIFY) .. 3

41. When you have to pay at the dentist does he usually tell you what the total cost is made up of?

Yes 1
No 2
Never paid 3

42. I'd like you to look at these different treatments and tell me how much you think each would cost, whether it would cost nothing or whether it would cost £2 or less, between £2 and £5, or £5 or more?

SHOW CARDS B AND C

COURSE OF TREATMENT (B)	TREATMENT WOULD COST				
	Nothing (Free)	£2 or less	Between £2 & £5	£5 or more	DK
Exam, 2 teeth out	1	2	3	4	5
Exam, 1 large filling, 1 tooth out	1	2	3	4	5
Examination only	1	2	3	4	5
Exam, 2 Xrays, scale and polish, 1 small filling	1	2	3	4	5
Exam, 4 teeth out, new dentures fitted	1	2	3	4	5
Exam, 2 Xrays, 6 teeth out, gas	1	2	3	4	5
Repair of cracked denture	1	2	3	4	5
Exam, 2 Xrays, scale and polish	1	2	3	4	5

13

45 People have mentioned all sorts of things that make them put off going to the dentist. Can you look at this card and tell me for each of the statements I read out whether these things apply to you very much, a fair amount, not very much or not at all.

SHOW CARD D

	APPLIES TO ME			
	very much	a fair amount	not very much	not at all	DK

I put off going to the dentist because ....

... I'm scared of the dentist ..	1 ...... 2 .... 3 .... 4 5
... It's difficult to get time off work	1 ...... 2 .... 3 .... 4 5
... I don't like having fillings	1 ...... 2 .... 3 .... 4 5
... It's too expensive to go too often	1 ...... 2 .... 3 .... 4 5
... I haven't got a regular dentist ...	1 ...... 2 .... 3 .... 4 5
... I can't be bothered really .	1 ...... 2 .... 3 .... 4 5
... Of the thought of having teeth out	1 ...... 2 .... 3 .... 4 5
.... It's difficult to get an appointment	1 ...... 2 .... 3 .... 4 5
It's a long way to go	1 ...... 2 .... 3 .... 4 5

46 What do you find most unpleasant about going to the dentist?

47 Are there any other comments you would like to make about your teeth or going to the dentist?

43 For most kinds of treatment under the National Health Service the patient pays the full cost up to the first £5

(a) As a maximum charge do you think £5 is

RUNNING PROMPT

too high 1
about right 2
or   too low? 3

(b) A few kinds of dental treatment are rather expensive and so the patient has to pay more than £5 to be treated under the National Health Service.

Do you know what kinds of treatment cost the patient more than £5?

Yes 1   ask (c)
No 2

IF YES (1)
(c) What kinds of treatment cost the patient more than £5?

44 Some people get exemption from dental charges so that all the treatment they have is free. Do you know what kinds of people get free treatment?

Yes 1   ask (a)
No 2

IF YES (1)
(a) What kinds of people get free treatment?

Pregnant or nursing mothers...... 1
Other (SPECIFY) 2

152 a) Grateful for their help - asking for a little more in order to complete the picture.

b) Some things only a dentist looking at your teeth would see.

c) Asking anybody who has some teeth if dentist can come back in a few days time.

d) He won't comment on your teeth at all, to you or anyone else (ethics).

e) Results will help to estimate the need for treatment.

f) Reassurance that it will not hurt at all, and interviewer will be there.

g) Length of time for examination.

Willing to have examination	1	see (h)
Not	2	see (j)

(h) IF WILLING (1)
    Appointment details

GIVE INFORMANT APPOINTMENT CARD

(j) IF NOT WILLING (2)
    NOTE COMMENTS

W559 OPCS 3/78

17

CLASSIFICATION - TO ALL

150 (a) Date of birth of informant

Day	Month	Year

(b) Sex of informant

Male	1
Female	2

(c) Age informant finished full time education

14 years or less	4
15 years.............	5
16 years	6
17 years	7
18 years or more	8
Still in f/t education	9

(d) Employment status of informant

Full time	1
Part time	2
Not in employment ...	3

(e) Marital status of informant

Married	1
Single	2
W/S/D	3

(f) What is the occupation of the informant?
(GIVE OCCUPATION AND INDUSTRY)

(g) IS THE INFORMANT HOH OR NOT?

Informant HOH	1	go to Q152
Not	2	go to Q151

151 What is the occupation of the HOH?
(GIVE OCCUPATION AND INDUSTRY)

16

89

S1112

Area No.	Address No.			Person

ADULT DENTAL HEALTH

UK 1978

Interview questionnaire 2

Has (Had) partial dentures

Interviewer's Name ....   Inf. ....

Interviewer's No. ....

I'd like to talk first about your natural teeth and how they are at the moment.

1. Many people suffer from toothache at one time or another. During the last four weeks have you had toothache at all or not?	Had toothache	1
	Not	2
2. During the last four weeks have you lost any fillings or have any bits broken off your teeth?	Fillings lost/tooth. broken ..	1
	None	2
3. Do you think any of your teeth are at all loose?	Some loose	1
	None	2
4. When you are eating or drinking are there any teeth that you avoid using?	Avoids some	1
	Does not	2 ask (a)
IF AVOIDS SOME (1) (a) What is the main reason for you avoiding those teeth?		
5. (Can I just check) do you think any of your teeth are decayed at the moment?	Teeth decayed	1
	Not	2

1

Dental health is not only to do with teeth but with gums as well

6. Are your gums swollen at all at the moment?
Gums swollen ... 1
Not 2

7 Are your gums inflamed, that is redder than usual, at the moment?
Gums inflamed 1
Not 2

8 During the last four weeks have your gums bled at all for example when you brushed your teeth or at any other time?
Gums bled 1
Have not 2
ask (a)

9 Do you have any other sort of trouble with your gums at the moment?
Other trouble 1
Not 2

IF OTHER TROUBLE (1)
(a) What other trouble do you have?

10 If you were to go to the dentist tomorrow do you think you would need any treatment or not?
Need treatment .. 1
Not 2
ask (a)

IF NEED TREATMENT (1)
(a) What sort of treatment do you think you would need?
PROMPT AS NEC.
CODE ALL THAT APPLY
Fillings 1
Extractions 2
Fillings/extractions but dk which ... 3
Other (SPECIFY) 4

11 (a) If you went to the dentist with an aching back tooth would you prefer the dentist to take it out or to fill it?
PROMPT AS NEC. "Supposing it could be filled"
Take it out ... 1
Fill it 2
Other (SPECIFY) ... 3

(b) If you went to the dentist with an aching front tooth would you prefer the dentist to take it out or to fill it?
PROMPT AS NEC. "Supposing it could be filled"
Take it out ... 1
Fill it 2
Other (SPECIFY) ... 3

2

12(a)   DNA

(b) A lot of people eventually have their own teeth out and have full dentures. Do you find the thought of losing all your own teeth and having full dentures ...
RUNNING PROMPT
.....very upsetting .. 1
a little upsetting .. 2
or not at all upsetting .. 3

13 Do you think at sometime you will have to have full dentures or do you think you will always keep some of your natural teeth?
Have full dentures ... 1
Keep natural teeth .. 2
D.K. 3
ask (a)

IF HAVE FULL DENTURES (1)
(a) At what age do you think you'll first need full dentures?
PROMPT AS NECESSARY
70's or more . 7
60's 6
50's 5
40's 4
30's 3
20's 2

14 Thinking of the people you know around your age about how many of them have full dentures; would you say it was ...
RUNNING PROMPT
All or most of them 1
Some of them 2
very few or none of them... 3

15 Whether or not teeth are lost is due partly to how healthy they are and different people have different ideas as to what things help to keep teeth healthy. I'd like to talk about some things people have mentioned. Can you tell me how important you consider them for keeping natural teeth healthy.
HAND OVER CARD A
Would you say that .....

	FOR KEEPING NATURAL TEETH HEALTHY				
	very important	fairly important	not very important	not at all important	D.K.
(i) Not eating sweets is ...	1	2	3	4	5
(ii) Regular visits to the dentist are	1	2	3	4	5
(iii) Cleaning teeth regularly is	1	2	3	4	5
(iv) Having fluoride in the water is	1	2	3	4	5

3

91

Now I'd like to talk a little about cleaning your natural teeth

16 (a) How often do you clean your teeth nowadays?

Never .... 9 [go to Q.17]
Once a day 1
Twice a day ... 2
More than twice a day ... 3
.......per............. Other (SPECIFY) 4

(b) At what time of the day do you clean them?

Before breakfast 1
After breakfast 2
Midday 3
Tea time 4
After evening meal 5
Last thing at night 6
Other (SPECIFY) 7

IF MORNING AND NO BREAKFAST RING 'AFTER BREAKFAST' (2)

(c) About how long ago did you start using the toothbrush you've got now? Was it ...

RUNNING PROMPT

less than 3 months 1
3 months, but less than 6 months .. 2
6 months, but less than a year 3
or a year or more ago? 4
D.K. 5
No toothbrush 6

(e) Do you use toothpaste, toothpowder or something else to clean your teeth?

Toothpaste ...... 1 ask (f)
Toothpowder 2
Other .... 3 ask (g)
(SPECIFY)

IF TOOTHPASTE OR TOOTHPOWDER (1 or 2)

(f) Thinking of the toothpaste (toothpowder) you use at the moment does it contain fluoride or not?

Contains fluoride . 1
Does not .... 2 ask (g)
Don't know 3

(g) (Can I just check) do you ever use anything else to clean your natural teeth such as dental floss or woodsticks?

Dental floss 1
Woodsticks 2
Other (SPECIFY) ... 3

4

Can I talk now about your childhood dental experiences

17 When you were a child how much encouragement were you given to clean your teeth? Were you given ....

RUNNING PROMPT

a great deal 1
a fair amount 2
not much 3
or no encouragement at all?.. 4

18 When you were a child (that is before you were 16) did you ever go to a dentist?

Went to a dentist .. 1 ask (a)
Did not .... 2 go to Q19

IF WENT TO A DENTIST (1)

(a) Did you go to the school dentist, to some other dentist or both?

School dentist ..... 1 ask (c)
Other dentist ...... 2 ask (b)
Both 3

IF WENT TO OTHER DENTIST OR BOTH (2),(3)

(b) (Excluding visits to the school dentist) as a child, did you go to the dentist for ...

a regular check up 1
an occasional check up .. 2 ask (c)
or only when you were having trouble with your teeth? .. 3
Other (SPECIFY) 4

(c) Thinking now about any treatment you had then. Did you have any teeth filled before you were 16?

Teeth filled 1
Not 2
DK/c n't remember .. 3

(d) Did you have any teeth taken out when you were that age?

Teeth taken out 1
Not 2
DK/can't remember .. 3

(e) Nowadays children sometimes have a brace fitted or teeth taken out to help straighten their teeth. Did you have any treatment to straighten or improve the appearance of your teeth?

Had treatment ..... 1 ask (f)
Did not 2
DK/can't remember .. 3

IF HAD TREATMENT (1)

(f) Did you have a brace fitted, teeth taken out, both of these or some other treatment?

Brace fitted 1
Teeth taken out 2
Both 3
Other (SPECIFY) ... 4

5

7

As well as treating people's teeth dentists can give advice to their patients on caring for their teeth and mouths and on preventing disease.

23 Has a dentist or any of his staff demonstrated to you the best way to clean your teeth?

Demonstrated 1   ask (a)
Not 2

IF DEMONSTRATED (1)
(a) Who was it who demonstrated teeth cleaning to you? Was it ...

... a dentist 1
a dental nurse or hygienist 2
RUNNING PROMPT
or somebody else (SPECIFY)? 3

24 Has a dentist or any of his staff ever given you any advice on caring for your gums?

Given advice 1   ask (a-b)
Not 2

IF GIVEN ADVICE (1)
(a) Who was it who gave you the advice? Was it ...

a dentist 1
a dental nurse or hygienist 2
RUNNING PROMPT
or somebody else (SPECIFY)? 3

(b) What advice did he/she give you?

25 Has a dentist or any of his staff ever advised you about eating sweets or other sugary things?

Advised 1   ask (a-b)
Not 2

IF ADVISED (1)
(a) Who was it who gave you the advice? Was it ...

a dentist 1
a dental nurse or hygienist 2
RUNNING PROMPT
or somebody else (SPECIFY)? 3

(b) What did he/she say?

We've talked a little about childhood and now I'd like to talk about the dental experiences you've had through the whole of your life.
IF TEETH FILLED WHEN CHILD (Q18(c) CODE (1)) RING (1) AND ASK (a-b)

19 Have you ever had any teeth filled?

Teeth filled 1   ask (a-b)
Not 2   Go to Q20

IF TEETH FILLED (1)
(a) Have you ever had an injection in your gum to kill the pain of a filling?

Injection in gum 1   ask (c)
Not 2

(b) Have you ever had an injection in your arm to kill the pain of a filling?

Injection in arm 1   ask (c)
Not 2   see (c)

IF HAD INJECTION (a) OR (b) CODE (1)
(c) Do you usually have an injection when you're having a filling done?

Usually 1
Not 2

IF TEETH TAKEN OUT WHEN CHILD (Q18 (d) CODE (1)) RING (1) AND ASK (a-c)

20 Have you ever had any teeth taken out?

Teeth taken out 1   ask (a-c)
Not 2   Go to Q21

IF TEETH TAKEN OUT (1)
(a) Have you ever had gas to have teeth taken out?

Had gas 1
Not 2

(b) Have you ever had an injection in your gum to have teeth taken out?

Injection in gum 1
Not 2

(c) Have you ever had an injection in your arm to have teeth taken out?

Injection in arm 1
Not 2

21 Have you ever had an Xray taken of your teeth?

Had Xray 1   ask (a)
Not 2

IF HAD XRAY (1)
(a) Do you usually have an Xray taken of your teeth when you go to the dentist?

Usually has Xray 1
Does not 2

22 The wisdom teeth, which are the very back teeth, often come through later than the other teeth and sometimes don't come through at all. Can you tell me which of your wisdom teeth have, at sometime, come through.
Has the one at the ... come through or not?

	top left	top right	bottom left	bottom right
Come through	1	1	1	1
Not come through	2	2	2	2
DK	3	3	3	3
still got it .	4	4	4	4
taken out	5	5	5	5

ask (a)

IF COME THROUGH (1)
(a) Have you still got the ... wisdom tooth or have you had it out since?

6

Another part of dentist's work is to provide treatment to improve the appearance of teeth which are crooked or protruding.

SHOW CARD A

26(a) How important do you think it is that children with crooked or protruding teeth should have them straightened. Do you think it is ..

	... very important	1
RUNNING	fairly important ...	2
PROMPT	not very important .	3
	or not at all important?	4

(b) How important do you think it is that adults with crooked or protruding teeth should have them straightened. Do you think it is ..

	... very important	1	
RUNNING	fairly important ...	2	see (c)
PROMPT	not very important .	3	
	or not at all important?	4	

IF ONE LESS IMPORTANT THAN OTHER

(c) Why do you think it is less important for ...... to have their teeth straightened?

27 How do you feel about your own teeth are you satisfied or not satisfied with the way they look?

Satisfied	1	go to Q28
Not satisfied	2	ask (a-b)
Informant says DNA ...	3	go to Q28

IF NOT SATISFIED (2)

(a) What is it about the way your teeth look that you're not satisfied with?

(b) Have you ever talked to a dentist about the appearance of your teeth?

Talked to dentist	1	ask (c)
Not	2	ask (d)

IF TALKED TO DENTIST (1)

(c) What did the dentist say?

IF NOT (2)

(d) Is there any reason why you haven't talked to a dentist about the appearance of your teeth?

8

I'd like to talk now about going to the dentist

28 Have you been to the dentist since the beginning of November (December) that's about six months ago?

Yes	1	ask (a)
No	2	ask (b)

IF YES (1)

(a) (Can I just check) are you in the middle of a course of treatment now or not?

In middle of treatment ..	1	go to Q29
Not	2	

IF NO (2)

(b) Have you been to the dentist since last April (May/June), that's about a year ago?

Yes	1	go to Q29
No	2	ask (c)

IF NO (b) CODE (2)

(c) About how long ago was your last visit to the dentist? PROMPT IF NEC.

More than 1 up to 2 years ago	1	ask (d)
More than 2 up to 3 years ago	2	go to Q29
More than 3 up to 5 years ago	3	
More than that (SPECIFY)	4	
Never	5	go to Q50

IF Q28(c) CODE (1)

(d) Was this before or after April 1st 1977.

Before April 1st	1
April 1st or after	2

29 The last time you went to the dentist what made you go? Was it because you were having some trouble with your teeth or for a check up or for some other reason?

Trouble with teeth .	1	ask (a)
Check up	2	
Other (SPECIFY)	3	

IF TROUBLE WITH TEETH (1)

(a) Did you have toothache or did you have some other trouble with your teeth?

Toothache	1
Other (SPECIFY)	2

30 When people go to the dentist for a check up or because they've got trouble with their teeth, they sometimes have to make more than one visit for the dentist to carry out any treatment they might need.
When you last went to the dentist how many visits did you have to make?

One visit	1
Two visits	2
Three visits	3
Four visits	4
Five or more	5

9

31 (Can I just check) during the visit(s) you made to the dentist for that course of treatment did you have any ...

	Yes	No	DK	
..... X rays taken	1	2	3	
Teeth filled	1	2	3	
Teeth taken out	1	2	3	
Teeth scaled (scraped, cleaned) and polished	1	2	3	
New dentures fitted	1	2	3	
Old dentures repaired	1	2	3	
Other treatment (SPECIFY)	1	2	3	

INDIVIDUAL PROMPT

First time ... 1   ask (c)
Been before .. 2   ask (a-b)

32 Was your treatment under the National Health Service, was it private or was it something else?

National Health Service	1	ask (b)
Private	2	ask (b)
N.H.S. and private	3	ask (a-b)
Community Dental Service	4	
Armed Forces	5	
Other (SPECIFY)	6	

IF N.H.S. AND PRIVATE (3)
(a) What treatment did you have privately?

IF ANY PRIVATE (2 or 3)
(b) What was the main reason for you having this treatment done privately?

33 How much did the treatment cost you?

Cost (SPECIFY)	1	ask (a)
Nothing	2	ask (b)
DK	3	go to Q34

IF PAID FOR TREATMENT (1)
(a) Did the treatment cost more than you expected, about what you expected or less than you expected?

More than expected	1	
About what expected	2	go to Q34
Less than expected	3	
Other (SPECIFY)	4	

IF NOTHING (2)
(b) Why didn't it cost you anything?

No treatment	1	go to Q34
Under 21, pregnant or nursing mother	2	
Other (SPECIFY)	3	ask (c)

(c) When you went to the dentist did you expect the treatment would be free?

Yes	1
No	2

10

34 Thinking about the dental practice you went to for your last treatment, was that the first time you had been to that dentist or group of dentists or had you been there before?

First time	1	ask (c)
Been before	2	ask (a-b)

IF BEEN BEFORE (2)
(a) For about how many years have you been going to that dentist or group of dentists?

Less than a year	1
One year less than two	2
Two years less than five	3
Five years or more	4
DK/can't remember	5

(b) Does the dentist send you a reminder when it is time to go for your next check up?

Sends reminder	1	Go to Q35
Does not	2	ask (c)

IF DOES NOT SEND REMINDER (2) OR FIRST TIME (1)
(c) When you make an appointment to see the dentist do you usually make it ....

... at the end of your previous treatment	1	go to Q35
some time before the date that you want the appointment	2	
or when you want to see the dentist as soon as possible	3	ask (d)
Other (SPECIFY)	4	go to Q35

IF CODE (2) OR (3)
(d) Last time you wanted to see the dentist about how long did you have to wait for an appointment?

35 How did you come to choose that particular dentist?

Can't remember 9

11

Page 13

I'd like to talk generally now about the cost of dental treatment under the National Health Service.

39. When you go to the dentist to have treatment do you normally have some idea of how much it's going to cost you?

Has some idea .. 1
Does not 2   ask (a)

40. Do you know where you can find out about National Health Service dental charges?

Yes 1
No 2

IF YES (1)
(a) Where can you find out?

Dentist 1
G.P.O. 2
Other (SPECIFY). 3

41. When you have to pay at the dentist does he usually tell you what the total cost is made up of?

Yes 1
No 2
Never paid 3

42. I'd like you to look at these different treatments and tell me how much you think each would cost, whether it would cost nothing or whether it would cost £2 or less, between £2 and £5, or £5 or more?

SHOW CARDS B AND C

COURSE OF TREATMENT (B)	TREATMENT WOULD COST (C)				
	Nothing (Free)	£2 or less	Between £2 & £5	£5 or more	DK
Exam, 2 teeth out	1	2	3	4	5
Exam, 1 large filling, 1 tooth out	1	2	3	4	5
Examination only	1	2	3	4	5
Exam, 2 Xrays, scale and polish, 1 small filling	1	2	3	4	5
Exam, 4 teeth out, new dentures fitted	1	2	3	4	5
Exam, 2 Xrays, 6 teeth out, gas	1	2	3	4	5
Repair of cracked denture	1	2	3	4	5
Exam, 2 Xrays, scale and polish	1	2	3	4	5

13

Page 12

36. In the last five years have you had any difficulty getting any treatment under the National Health Service?

Had difficulty .. 1
Not 2   ask (a-b)
Not tried 3

IF HAD DIFFICULTY (1)
(a) What treatment couldn't you get?

ALL OF IT/
PART OF IT
IF PART WHAT PART?

(b) What did you do about it?

37. In general do you go to the dentist for ...

.. a regular check up 1   go to Q38
an occasional check up 2
or only when you're having trouble with your teeth .. 3   ask (a-b)

IF DOES NOT GO FOR A REGULAR CHECK UP (2 or 3)
(a) What is the main reason for you not going for a regular check up?

(b) (You've told me the main reason for you not going for a regular check up) now I'd like to ask about the kinds of circumstances when you would go to the dentist.
Would you go to the dentist if you had ....

	YES	NO
Occasional twinges of toothache	1	2
A tooth which felt loose	1	2
Not been to the dentist for a long time	1	2
A swollen face	1	2
Sore gums	1	2
A problem with your denture	1	2
Toothache which kept you awake at night	1	2
A gumboil	1	2
A tooth with a piece broken off	1	2
Gums which bled occasionally	1	2

38. Would you say that nowadays you go to the dentist more often, about the same or less often than you did five years ago?

More often 1   ask (a)
About the same .. 2
Less often 3   ask (a)

IF MORE OR LESS OFTEN (1 or 3)
(a) What has made you go more (less) often?

12

43 For most kinds of treatment under the National Health Service the patient pays the full cost up to the first £5

(a) As a maximum charge do you think £5 is.. ..too high 1
RUNNING   about right 2
PROMPT   or too low? 3

(b) A few kinds of dental treatment are rather expensive and so the patient has to pay more than £5 to be treated under the National Health Service.

Do you know what kinds of treatment cost the patient more than £5?

Yes .... 1 — ask (c)
No 2

IF YES (1)
(c) What kinds of treatment cost the patient more than £5?

44 Some people get exemption from dental charges so that all the treatment they have is free.
Do you know what kinds of people get free treatment?

Yes .... 1 — ask (a)
No 2

IF YES (1)
(a) What kinds of people get free treatment?

Pregnant or nursing mothers 1
Other (SPECIFY) 2

14

---

45 People have mentioned all sorts of things that make them put off going to the dentist. Can you look at this card and tell me for each of the statements I read out whether these things apply to you very much, a fair amount, not very much or not at all.

SHOW CARD D

I put off going to the dentist because ......

| | APPLIES TO ME | | | |
very much	a fair amount	not very much	not at all	DK
... I'm scared of the dentist ... 1	2	3	4	5
... It's difficult to get time off work 1	2	3	4	5
... I don't like having fillings 1	2	3	4	5
... It's too expensive to go too often ... 1	2	3	4	5
... I haven't got a regular dentist ... 1	2	3	4	5
... I can't be bothered really ... 1	2	3	4	5
... Of the thought of having teeth out 1	2	3	4	5
... It's difficult to get an appointment 1	2	3	4	5
... It's a long way to go 1	2	3	4	5

46 What do you find most unpleasant about going to the dentist?

47

DNA

15

I would like to talk now about your partial dentures (false teeth)

50(a) Have you ever had a top plate?

Has (had) top plate .	1	
Not	2	ask(d)

(b) Have you ever had a bottom plate?

Has (had) bottom plate 1	
Not 2	

ASK FOR EACH PLATE AS APPROPRIATE

		TOP PLATE	BOTTOM PLATE
(c) Is the top plate (bottom plate) a full plate or not?	Full plate .	1	1
	Not	2	2
IF NOT (2)			
(d) Has the top plate (bottom plate) got some front teeth on it, or is it all back teeth?	Some front .	1	1
	All back ...	2	2

51 DNA

(People with dentures sometimes get on better with one plate than the other so I'd like to talk about your top and bottom plates separately)

		TOP PLATE	BOTTOM PLATE	
52 Have you worn your top plate (bottom plate) at all during the last four weeks?	Yes, worn .	1	1	
	Not	2*	2*	ask (a-c)
IF WORN IN LAST FOUR WEEKS (1)				
(a) (Sometimes people don't get on very well with a new denture and go back to wearing their old one)				
Is the top plate (bottom plate) that you wear now the most recent one you've had or not?	Wears most recent.	8	8	
	Wears old one	9	9	
(I'd like to talk about the denture you wear)				
(b) Do you usually keep your top plate (bottom plate) in at night?	In at night	3	3	
	Not	4	4	
(c) Do you wear your top plate (bottom plate) from the time you get up to when you go to bed?	All daytime ..	5	5	
	Not	6*	6*	

SUBJECT CHANGE FROM

NATURAL TEETH TO

DENTURES

INTERVIEWER

FOR PLATES NOT WORN IN LAST FOUR WEEKS (2) ASK Q'S 53-54

FOR PLATES NOT WORN ALL DAYTIME (6) ASK Q'S 55-56

FOR PLATES WORN ALL DAYTIME (5) ASK Q'S 57-62

FOR PLATES WORN ALL DAYTIME Q52 CODE (5)

Some people are fortunate with the fit of their dentures while others are not

		TOP PLATE	BOTTOM PLATE	
57	Do you have any difficulties with your top plate (bottom plate) when you yawn?			
	Difficulties	1*	1*	
	Not	2	2	
58	Do you have any difficulties with your top plate (bottom plate) when you are talking?			
	Difficulties	1*	1*	
	Not	2	2	
59	Would you have any difficulties with your top plate (bottom plate) if you were chewing meat?			
	Difficulties	1*	1*	
	Not	2	2	
60	Would you have any difficulties with your top plate (bottom plate) if you were to bite into a raw apple?			
	Difficulties	1*	1*	
	No	2	2	
61	During the last four weeks has your top plate (bottom plate) hurt or made your mouth sore or not?			
	Hurt/sore	1*	1*	
	Not	2	2	
62	Would you say that your top plate (bottom plate) is .... RUNNING PROMPT			
	... too loose	1*	1*	
	about right	2	2	
	or too tight?	3*	3*	

INTERVIEWER CHECK Q52 AND ABOVE

63	AT LEAST ONE CODE WITH AN ASTERISK RINGED	1	ask Q64
	NO CODES WITH AN ASTERISK RINGED	2	Go to Q65

64	You've said .... Are you planning to visit the dentist to see about your denture(s) for that or any other reason?		
	Planning to visit	1	
	Not	2	ask(a)

IF NOT (2)
(a) Is there any reason why you aren't planning to visit the dentist?

FOR PLATES NOT WORN IN LAST FOUR WEEKS Q52 CODE (2)

		TOP PLATE	BOTTOM PLATE	
53	Have you still got your top plate (bottom plate)?			
	Still got ..	1	1	ask(a)
	Not	2	2	ask(b)
	IF STILL GOT (1)			
	(a) Why don't you wear your top plate (bottom plate)?			
	Denture replaced with fixed appliance ..	1	1	go to Q150
	IF NOT (2)			
	(b) What happened to your top plate (bottom plate)?			
	Denture replaced with fixed appliance ..	1	1	go to Q150
54	Have you ever had a top plate (bottom plate) that you could wear?			
	Had plate ..	1	1	CHECK OTHER PLATE GO TO Q63 FOR THIS PLATE
	Not	2	2	

FOR PLATES WORN ALL DAYTIME Q52 CODE (6)

		TOP PLATE YES	TOP PLATE NO	BOTTOM PLATE YES	BOTTOM PLATE NO
55	Do you usually wear your top plate (bottom plate) when you				
	go out	1	2	1	2
	are eating	1	2	1	2
	INDIVIDUAL PROMPT are about the house .	1	2	1	2

56	Why don't you wear your top plate (bottom plate) all the time?	TOP PLATE	BOTTOM PLATE	
				CHECK OTHER PLATE GO TO Q63 FOR THIS PLATE

TO PEOPLE WHO HAVE WORN ONE OR BOTH PLATES IN LAST 4 WEEKS

NO PLATE WORN IN LAST 4 WEEKS   DNA ... X   Go to Q69

I'd like to talk now about cleaning dentures (false teeth)

65(a) Do you find that it is difficult to keep false teeth clean or not?
- Yes .. 1
- No ... 2

(b) How often do you clean your false teeth?

(c) Do you clean your false teeth by ...
INDIVIDUAL PROMPT

	Yes	No	
... Soaking them	1	2	see (d)
Brushing them	3	4	see (e)
Some other method . (SPECIFY)	5	6	

(d) IF YES, SOAKING THEM (1)
What do you soak them in?

(e) IF YES, BRUSHING THEM (3)
What do you brush them with?

66 Do you use anything to help keep your top plate (bottom plate) in place?

	TOP PLATE	BOTTOM PLATE	
Uses something ..	1	1	
Does not	2	2	ask (a)

(a) IF USES SOMETHING (1)
What do you use?

67 During the last four weeks have you put anything on your dentures or gums to prevent or ease soreness?
- Yes .. 1
- No ... 2

68 During the last four weeks have you taken any tablets or lozenges to ease soreness?
- Yes .. 1
- No ... 2

TO ALL WHO HAVE EVER HAD DENTURES

	TOP PLATE	BOTTOM PLATE	
69 How long ago did you get your present top plate (bottom plate)?			
Less than a year	1	1	
1 year, less than 2 years	2	2	
2 years, less than 5 years ...	3	3	
5 years, less than 10 years ...	4	4	
10 years, less than 20 years ..	5	5	
20 years, or more	6	6	

IF LOST ASK ABOUT THE PLATE THAT IS NOW LOST

70 Did you get your present top plate (bottom plate) through the National Health Service or did you pay for if privately?			
N.H.S	1	1	
Private	2	2	
Before N.H.S.	3	3	
Other (SPECIFY)	4	4	

(a) IF PRIVATE (2)
What was the main reason for you getting your top plate (bottom plate) privately?   ask (a)

71 DNA

72

73 Thinking about your present dentures
    how satisfied are (were) you with
    their appearance; are (were) you ...

... very satisfied	1	go to Q74
RUNNING	fairly satisfied	2	ask (a)
PROMPT	not very satisfied	3	
	or not at all satisfied? ...	4	
	Informant says DNA	5	go to Q74

(a) IF CODE (2, 3 or 4)
     You say you are (were) ..... rather than
     very satisfied. What is it about their appearance
     that you are (were) not completely satisfied with?

INTERVIEWER OBSERVE:
IF INFORMANT IS NOT WEARING TEETH AT TIME OF INTERVIEW – DNA 5   go to Q83

74(a) Some people who wear dentures
       don't like their family to see
       them without their teeth.
       How much does this worry you:
       very much, to some extent or
       not at all?

Very much	1
To some extent ..	2
Not at all	3
No family	4

(b) If people other than the family
     were to see you without your teeth
     how much would this worry you:
     very much, to some extent or
     not at all?

Very much	1
To some extent ..	2
Not at all	3

22

Questions 75 – 82 DNA

23

83 When you first had dentures fitted
did the dentist give you any advice
on how to chew with dentures?

Advice on chewing ..	1
None	2
Can't remember	3

84 Did the dentist give you any
advice on how to bite with the
front teeth of your dentures?

Advice on biting ...	1
None	2
Can't remember	3
Informant says DNA	4

85 Did the dentist talk to you at all
about the length of time it would take
you to get used to your dentures?

Yes, talked	1	ask (a)
Did not	2	
Can't remember	3	

IF YES, TALKED (1)
(a) How long did he say it would take
you to get used to them?

86 Did the dentist tell you how long
you should expect your dentures
to last?

Yes	1
No	2
Can't remember	3

87 When you first had your dentures
did the dentist or any of his staff
tell you how to clean them?

Yes, told	1
No	2
Can't remember	3

88 Did the dentist advise you about
wearing your dentures at night?

Advised	1	ask (a)
Did not	2	
Can't remember	3	

IF ADVISED (1)
(a) Did he advise you to keep them in
at night or to take them out?

Keep them in	1
Take them out	2
Other (SPECIFY)	3

89 Would you have liked the dentist to
have given you some (more) advice
on managing dentures?

Liked (more) advice	1
Would not	2

90 (Can I just check) when you first
had dentures fitted did the dentist
or any of his staff give you a leaflet
about wearing dentures?

Given leaflet	1
Not	2
Can't remember	3

91 When you first had partial dentures about how long
did it take you to get used to having them?

92 Coping with new dentures is always
strange at first. Was there anything
in particular about wearing
dentures that you hadn't expected?

Something unexpected .	1	ask (a)
Not	2	

IF SOMETHING UNEXPECTED (1)
(a) What was it?

93 Since you've had partial dentures
have you enjoyed your food ...
RUNNING
PROMPT

... more than before	1
about the same as before .	2
or less than before you had them?.	3

94 Since you've had partial dentures have
you had to change the kind of food
you eat?

Had to change	1	ask (a-b)
Not	2	

IF HAD TO CHANGE (1)
(a) What can you eat now that you
couldn't eat before?

Nothing	1

(b) What could you eat before
that you can't eat now?

Nothing	1

95 Since having partial dentures have you had any trouble with your natural teeth which you feel is connected with having dentures?

Had trouble 1   ask (a)
Not 2

IF HAD TROUBLE (1)
(a) What trouble have you had?

DNA

96 DNA

97 If you knew someone who thought they might soon have to have a partial denture for the first time what advice would you give them?

DNA

98

99 Since you first had dentures how many top plates (bottom plates) have you had altogether?

	TOP PLATE	BOTTOM PLATE
One plate only ..	1	1
Number _____		

IF MORE THAN ONE TOP PLATE (BOTTOM PLATE)
(a) When you had false teeth for the first time what combination of dentures did you have: a top plate only, a bottom plate only or both?

Top plate only 1
Bottom plate only .. 2
Both 3   ask (a–b)

(b) Was your first top plate (bottom plate) a full plate or not?

	TOP PLATE	BOTTOM PLATE
Full plate	1	1
Partial	2	2

IF PARTIAL (2)
(c) Did the top plate (bottom plate) have some front teeth on it or were they all back teeth?

	TOP PLATE	BOTTOM PLATE
Some front teeth .	1	1
All back teeth ..	2	2 ask (c)

26

100 How old were you when you first had some false teeth?

Age in years ....

101 Were your first false teeth mainly for the sake of appearance or mainly to help you to eat?

Mainly for sake of appearance . 1
Mainly to help you to eat 2

147 Since you had your first set of dentures how many more of your own teeth have you lost?

Number lost ....

TO PEOPLE WHO HAVE HAD MORE THAN ONE TOP PLATE (BOTTOM PLATE)(SEE Q99)

DNA: One plate only X   GO TO Q.149

148 You say you've had .... top plates (bottom plates). Were any of the top plate (bottom plate) replacements needed because ....

	TOP PLATE		BOTTOM PLATE	
	YES	NO/DK	YES	NO/DK
INDIVIDUAL PROMPT				
....(i) you'd had more teeth taken out	1	2	1	2
(ii) the previous plate hurt or caused ulcers ..	1	2	1	2
(iii) the previous plate was worn down, damaged or broken	1	2	1	2
(iv) the previous plate didn't fit properly....	1	2	1	2
(v) the previous plate didn't look right	1	2	1	2
(vi) the previous plate didn't match the other plate	1	2	1	2
(vii) other (SPECIFY)......				

149 Are there any other comments you would like to make about your teeth or dentures?

27

103

CLASSIFICATION - TO ALL

150 (a) Date of birth of informant

Day	Month	Year

(b) Sex of informant

Male 1
Female 2

(c) Age informant finished full time education

14 years or less .. 4
15 years 5
16 years 6
17 years 7
18 years or more .. 8
Still in f/t education ... 9

(d) Employment status of informant

Full time 1
Part time 2
Not in employment .. 3

(e) Marital status of informant

Married 1
Single 2
W/S/D 3

(f) What is the occupation of the informant?
(GIVE OCCUPATION AND INDUSTRY)

(g) IS THE INFORMANT HOH OR NOT?

Informant HOH 1   go to Q 152
Not 2   go to Q 151

151 What is the occupation of the HOH?
(GIVE OCCUPATION AND INDUSTRY)

INTRODUCE AS NECESSARY

152 a) Grateful for their help - asking for a little more in order to complete the picture.

b) Some things only a dentist looking at your teeth would see.

c) Asking anybody who has some teeth if dentist can come back in a few days time.

d) He won't comment on your teeth at all, to you or anyone else (ethics).

e) Results will help to estimate the need for treatment.

f) Reassurance that it will not hurt at all, and interviewer will be there.

g) Length of time for examination.

Willing to have examination 1   see (h)
Not 2   see (j)

IF WILLING (1)
(h) Appointment details

GIVE INFORMANT APPOINTMENT CARD

IF NOT WILLING(2)
(j) NOTE COMMENTS

W559 OPCS 3/78

S1112

Area No.	Address No.	Person

ADULT DENTAL HEALTH

UK 1978

Interview questionnaire 3

People with no natural teeth

Interviewer's Name ....

Interviewer's No. ....

Inf. ....

51 Could I just check, have you ever had a full set of dentures or not?

Have (had) full dentures . 1 ask(a)

Not 2

IF NOT (2)
(a) Why have you never had full dentures?

GO TO Q 75

52 People with full dentures sometimes get on better with one plate than the other so I'd like to talk about your top and bottom plates separately.

	TOP PLATE	BOTTOM PLATE
Have you worn your top plate (bottom plate) at all during the last four weeks?		
Yes, worn ..	1	1
Not	2*	2*
		ask(a-c)
IF WORN IN LAST FOUR WEEKS (1)		
(a) (Sometimes people don't get on very well with a new denture and go back to wearing their old one).		
Is the top plate (bottom plate) that you wear now the most recent one you've had or not?		
Wears most recent .	8	8
Wears old one	9	9
(I'd like to talk about the denture you wear)		
(b) Do you usually keep your top plate (bottom plate) in at night?		
In at night	3	3
Not	4	4
(c) Do you wear your top plate (bottom plate) from the time you get up to when you go to bed?		
All daytime	5	5
Not	6*	6*

INTERVIEWER

FOR PLATES NOT WORN IN LAST FOUR WEEKS (2) ASK Q'S 53-54

FOR PLATES NOT WORN ALL DAYTIME (6) ASK Q's 55-56

FOR PLATES WORN ALL DAYTIME (5) ASK Q's 57-62

1

FOR PLATES WORN ALL DAYTIME Q52 CODE (5)

Some people are fortunate with the fit of their dentures while others are not

		TOP PLATE	BOTTOM PLATE	
57	Do you have any difficulties with your top plate (bottom plate) when you yawn?			
	Difficulties ..	1*	1*	
	Not	2	2	
58	Do you have any difficulties with your top plate (bottom plate) when you are talking?			
	Difficulties ..	1*	1*	
	Not	2	2	
59	Would you have any difficulties with your top plate (bottom plate) if you were chewing meat?			
	Difficulties ..	1*	1*	
	Not	2	2	
60	Would you have any difficulties with your top plate (bottom plate) if you were to bite into a raw apple?			
	Difficulties ..	1*	1*	
	Not	2	2	
61	During the last four weeks has your top plate (bottom plate) hurt or made your mouth sore or not?			
	Hurt/sore	1*	1*	
	Not	2	2	
62	Would you say that your top plate (bottom plate) is .... RUNNING PROMPT			
	... too loose	1*	1*	
	about right ...	2	2	
	or too tight?	3*	3*	

INTERVIEWER CHECK Q52 AND ABOVE

63	AT LEAST ONE CODE WITH AN ASTERISK RINGED	1	ask Q64
	NO CODES WITH AN ASTERISK RINGED	2	Go to Q65

64	You've said .... Are you planning to visit the dentist to see about your dentures for that or any other reason?		
	Planning to visit	1	
	Not	2	ask(a)

IF NOT (2)
(a) Is there any reason why you aren't planning to visit the dentist?

3

FOR PLATES NOT WORN IN LAST FOUR WEEKS Q52 CODE (2)

		TOP PLATE	BOTTOM PLATE	
53	Have you still got your top plate (bottom plate)?			
	Still got..	1	1	ask(a)
	Not	2	2	ask(b)

IF STILL GOT (1)
(a) Why don't you wear your top plate (bottom plate)?

IF NOT (2)
(b) What happened to your top plate (bottom plate)?

		TOP PLATE	BOTTOM PLATE	
54	Have you ever had a full top plate (bottom plate) that you could wear?			
	Had plate	1	1	
	Not	2	2	CHECK OTHER PLATE GO TO Q63 FOR THIS PLATE

FOR PLATES NOT WORN ALL DAYTIME Q52 CODE (6)

		TOP PLATE YES	TOP PLATE NO	BOTTOM PLATE YES	BOTTOM PLATE NO
55	Do you usually wear your top plate (bottom plate) when you				
	go out	1	2	1	2
	are eating	1	2	1	2
INDIVIDUAL PROMPT	are about the house	1	2	1	2

	TOP PLATE	BOTTOM PLATE	
56 Why don't you wear your top plate (bottom plate) all the time?			CHECK OTHER PLATE GO TO Q63 FOR THIS PLATE

2

106

Page 4

TO PEOPLE WHO HAVE WORN ONE OR BOTH PLATES IN LAST 4 WEEKS

NEITHER PLATE WORN IN LAST 4 WEEKS   DNA ...   X   Go to Q69

I'd like to talk now about cleaning dentures (false teeth)

65(a) Do you find that it is difficult to keep false teeth clean or not?

Yes 1
No 2

(b) How often do you clean your false teeth?

....

(c) Do you clean your false teeth by ....

		Yes	No	
INDIVIDUAL PROMPT	... Soaking them	1	2	see (d)
	Brushing them	3	4	see (e)
	Some other method ... (SPECIFY)	5	6	

IF YES, SOAKING THEM (1)
(d) What do you soak them in?

IF YES, BRUSHING THEM (3)
(e) What do you brush them with?

66 Do you use anything to help keep your top plate (bottom plate) in place?

	TOP PLATE	BOTTOM PLATE	
Uses something ..	1	1	
Does not	2	2	ask(a)

IF USES SOMETHING (1)
(a) What do you use?

67 During the last four weeks have you put anything on your dentures or gums to prevent or ease soreness?

Yes 1
No 2

68 During the last four weeks have you taken any tablets or lozenges to ease soreness?

Yes 1
No 2

4

Page 5

TO ALL WHO HAVE EVER HAD DENTURES

	TOP PLATE	BOTTOM PLATE

69 How long ago did you get your present top plate (bottom plate)?

	TOP PLATE	BOTTOM PLATE
Less than a year	1	1
1 year, less than 2 years ..	2	2
2 years, less than 5 years .	3	3
5 years, less than 10 years	4	4
10 years, less than 20 yrs .	5	5
20 years, or more	6	6

IF LOST ASK ABOUT THE PLATE THAT IS NOW LOST

70 Did you get your present top plate (bottom plate) through the National Health Service or did you pay for it privately?

	TOP PLATE	BOTTOM PLATE	
N.H.S...........	1	1	
Private	2	2	
Before N.H.S. ..	3	3	
Other (SPECIFY) .	4	4	ask(a)

IF PRIVATE (2)
(a) What was the main reason for you getting your top plate (bottom plate) privately?

71 Do you know how much it would cost you nowadays to have a full set of false teeth under the National Health Service?

Yes	1	
No	2	ask (a)

IF YES (1)
(a) How much does it cost?

5

(Questions 75–82)

TO ALL
I'd like to talk now about when you had the last of your natural teeth out

75 How many years ago did you have the last of your own teeth taken out?

PROMPT AS NECESSARY

Up to 5 years ago	1
Over 5 up to 10 years ago	2
Over 10 up to 15 years ago	3
Over 15 up to 20 years ago	4
Over 20 up to 30 years ago	5
Over 30 years ago	6 → ask(a)

IF OVER 30 YEARS AGO (6)
(a) Was this before or after 1948 when the National Health Service began?

Before	1
After	2

76 How old were you when you lost the last of your natural teeth?

AGE IN YEARS

77 When you lost the last of your own teeth how many teeth were there to be taken out altogether?

1 – 11	1
12 – 20	2
21 or more	3

IF ONLY ONE TOOTH TAKEN OUT RING CODE (1)

78 Were these all taken out together or were they taken out over a series of visits?

All in one visit ...	1
Series of visits ..	2

79 Why did the last of your own teeth have to be taken out, was it because....

CODE ALL THAT APPLY

... the teeth were decayed ..	1
the gums were bad	2
or was it for some other reason (SPECIFY)?.........	3

80 Did you find losing the last of your natural teeth and having full dentures

very upsetting	1
a little upsetting	2
or not at all upsetting? .	3

81 Did you suggest to the dentist that the last of your natural teeth should come out or did he suggest this to you?

Informant suggested to dentist .	1
Dentist suggested to informant .	2
Other (SPECIFY)	3

TO ALL WHO HAVE EVER HAD FULL DENTURES Q51 (1)
DNA: NEVER HAD FULL DENTURES ..X

82 How long after you had the last of your own teeth out did you have false teeth in, was it ...

RUNNING PROMPT

the same day	1
up to 1 month	2
more than 1 month up to 3 months .	3
more than 3 months up to 6 months .	4
or more than 6 months later?	5

Go to Q.95

(Questions 72–74)

72 How many full top plates (bottom plates) have you had since the last of your natural teeth were taken out?

	TOP PLATE	BOTTOM PLATE	
1	1	1	
2	2	2	
3	3	3	
4	4	4	
5 or more ...	5	5	go to Q.73

IF 2 OR MORE (2,3,4 or 5)
(a) Were any of your top plate (bottom plate) replacements needed because the previous plate .....

I M P R O V E D   U P L A T

	TOP PLATE YES	TOP PLATE NO/DK	BOTTOM PLATE YES	BOTTOM PLATE NO/DK	
(i) hurt or caused ulcers	..1	..2 ..	..1	..2 ..	
(ii) was worn down, damaged or broken ..	..1	..2 ..	..1	..2 ..	
(iii) didn't fit properly	..1	..2 ..	..1	..2 ..	
(iv) didn't look right	..1	..2 ..	..1	..2 ..	
(v) didn't match the other plate	..1	..2 ..	..1	..2 ..	
(vi) other (SPECIFY)	..1	..2 ..	..1	..2 ..	ask(a)

73 Thinking about your present dentures how satisfied are (were) you with their appearance; are (were) you ....

RUNNING PROMPT

...very satisfied	1
fairly satisfied	2
not very satisfied ..	3
or not at all satisfied? ..	4

IF CODE (2, 3 or 4)
(a) You say you are (were) .... rather than very satisfied. What is it about their appearance that you are (were) not completely satisfied with?

INTERVIEWER OBSERVE:
IF INFORMANT IS NOT WEARING TEETH AT TIME OF INTERVIEW – DNA .... 5 → Go to Q.75

74 (a) Some people who wear dentures don't like their family to see them without their teeth. How much does this worry you: very much, to some extent or not at all?

Very much	1
To some extent .	2
Not at all	3
No family	4

(b) If people other than the family were to see you without your teeth how much would this worry you: very much, to some extent or not at all?

Very much	1
To some extent .	2
Not at all	3

DNA: TEETH TAKEN OUT MORE THAN TEN YEARS AGO   X   Go to Q.95

83 When you first had full dentures did the dentist give you any advice on how to chew with dentures?

Advice on chewing	1
None	2
Can't remember	3

84 Did the dentist give you any advice on how to bite with the front teeth of your dentures?

Advice on biting	1
None	2
Can't remember	3

85 Did the dentist talk to you at all about the length of time it would take you to get used to your dentures?

Yes, talked	1 ask(a)
Did not	2
Can't remember	3

IF YES, TALKED (1)
(a) How long did he say it would take you to get used to them?

86 Did the dentist tell you how long you should expect your dentures to last?

Yes	1
No	2
Can't remember	3

87 When you first had full dentures did the dentist or any of his staff tell you how to clean them?

Yes, told	1
No	2
Can't remember	3

88 Did the dentist advise you about wearing your dentures at night?

Advised	1 ask(a)
Did not	2
Can't remember	3

IF ADVISED (1)
(a) Did he advise you to keep them in at night or to take them out?

Keep them in	1
Take them out	2
Other (SPECIFY)	3

89 Would you have liked the dentist to have given you some (more) advice on managing dentures?

Liked(more)advice	1
Would not	2

90 (Can I just check) when you first had full dentures did the dentist or any of his staff give you a leaflet about wearing full dentures?

Given leaflet	1
Not	2
Can't remember	3

8

---

91 When you first had full dentures about how long did it take you to get used to having them?

92 Coping with new dentures is always strange at first. Was there anything in particular about wearing full dentures that you hadn't expected?

Something unexpected	1 ask(a)
Not	2

IF SOMETHING UNEXPECTED (1)
(a) What was it?

93 Since you've had full dentures have you enjoyed your food .....

... more than before	1
about the same as before	2
or less than before you had them	3

94 Since you've had full dentures have you had to change the kind of food you eat?

Had to change	1 ask(a-b)
Not	2

IF HAD TO CHANGE (1)
(a) What can you eat now that you couldn't eat before?

Nothing	1

(b) What could you eat before that you can't eat now?

Nothing	1

9

TO ALL

95 Thinking about when you lost the last of your natural teeth can you tell me a little more about how you felt?

96 Did you expect to lose your teeth around then or were you surprised to have them out at that age?

Expected to lose	1
Surprised at that age ...	2
Other (SPECIFY)	3

97 If you knew someone who thought they might soon have to have the rest of their teeth out and full dentures fitted what advice would you give them?

(We've been talking about full dentures but, of course) people may have partial dentures (some false teeth) before they lose all their own teeth.

98 When you had the last of your own teeth out had you previously had any dentures?

Previously had dentures ..	1	ask(a)
Did not	2	go to Q.115

IF PREVIOUSLY HAD DENTURES(1)

(a) What kind of dentures did you have, a top plate only, a bottom plate only or both?

Top plate only ...	1	ask(b)
Bottom plate only.	2	ask(c)
Both	3	ask(b-c)

IF TOP PLATE OR BOTH (1 or 3)

(b) Was the top plate a full plate or not?

Full top plate ...	1
Partial	2

IF BOTTOM PLATE OF BOTH (2 or 3)

(c) Was the bottom plate a full-plate or not?

Full bottom plate.	1
Partial	2

99 [Was that top plate (bottom plate)] Were those plates the only partial denture(s) you'd had or had you previously had other dentures?

One set only	1	Go to Q.100
Had others	2	ask(a)

IF HAD OTHERS (2)

(a) When you had dentures for the very first time what did you have a top plate only, a bottom plate only or both?

Top plate only ...	1	ask(b)
Bottom plate only.	2	ask(c)
Both	3	ask(b-c)

IF TOP PLATE OR BOTH (1 or 3)

(b) Was the top plate a full plate or not?

Full top plate ...	1
Partial	2

IF BOTTOM PLATE OR BOTH (2 or 3)

(c) Was the bottom plate a full plate or not?

Full bottom plate.	1
Partial	2

100 How old were you when you first had some false teeth?

Age in years	

101 Were your first false teeth mainly for the sake of appearance or mainly to help you to eat?

Mainly for sake of appearance .	1
Mainly to help you to eat	2

TO ALL

115 Different people have different ideas as to what things help to keep teeth healthy. I'd like to talk to you about some things people have mentioned. Can you tell me how important you consider them for keeping natural teeth healthy?

SHOW CARD A

	FOR KEEPING NATURAL TEETH HEALTHY				
Would you say that	very important	fairly important	not very important	not at all important	DK
(i) Not eating sweets is	1	2	3	4	5
(ii) Regular visits to the dentist are	1	2	3	4	5
(iii) Cleaning teeth regularly is	1	2	3	4	5
(iv) Having fluoride in the water is	1	2	3	4	5

116 DNA

SUBJECT CHANGE FROM
DENTURES TO
GENERAL DENTAL EXPERIENCES

I'd like to talk now about your childhood dental experiences

117 When you were a child how much encouragement were you given to clean your teeth. Were you given ...

RUNNING PROMPT

a great deal 1
a fair amount 2
not much 3
or no encouragement at all. 4

118 When you were a child (that is before you were 16) did you ever go to a dentist?

Went to a dentist. 1   ask(a)
Did not 2   Go to Q.119

(a) IF WENT TO A DENTIST (1)
Did you go to the school dentist some other dentist or both?

School dentist ... 1   ask(c-d)
Other dentist 2
Both 3   ask(b-d)

(b) IF OTHER DENTIST OR BOTH (2 or 3)
(Excluding visits to the school dentist) as a child did you go to the dentist for ....

RUNNING PROMPT

a regular check up 1
an occasional check up .. 2
or only when you were having trouble with your teeth?. 3
Other (SPECIFY) 4

(c) Thinking about any treatment you had then
Did you have any teeth filled before you were 16?

Teeth filled 1
Not 2
DK/can't remember. 3

(d) Did you have any teeth taken out before you were 16?

Teeth taken out 1
Not 2
DK/Can't remember. 3

13

12

111

I'd like to talk now about going to the dentist.

128 Have you been to the dentist in the last year?

Yes	1	ask (a)
No	2	ask (b)

(a) IF YES (1)
(Can I just check) are you in the middle of a course of treatment now or not?

In middle of treatment .	1	go to Q129
Not	2	

(b) IF NO (2)
About how long ago was your last visit to the dentist?

PROMPT AS NECESSARY

More than 1 up to 2 years ago	1	ask (d)
More than 2 up to 3 years ago	2	go to Q129
More than 3 up to 5 years ago	3	
More than 5 up to 10 years ago	4	
More than 10 up to 15 years ago	5	go to Q145
More than 15 up to 20 years ago	6	
More than 20 years ago	7	ask (c)

(c) IF LAST WENT TO DENTIST MORE THAN 20 YEARS AGO (7)
Was your last visit to the dentist since 1948 or before 1948?

1948 or since	1	go to Q145
Before 1948...............	2	

(d) IF MORE THAN 1 UP TO 2 YEARS AGO (b) CODE (1)
Was your last visit before or after April 1st 1977?

Before April 1st	1
April 1st or after	2

129 The last time you went to the dentist what was it that made you go?

130 For the treatment you needed at that time how many visits did you have to make to the dentist?

One visit............	1
Two visits	2
Three visits	3
Four visits..........	4
Five or more visits....	5

15

(We've talked a little about childhood and) now I'd like to talk about the dental experiences you've had through the whole of your life

IF TEETH FILLED WHEN CHILD (Q118 (c) CODE (1)) RING (1) AND ASK (a-b)

119 Have you ever had any teeth filled?

Teeth filled	1	ask(a-b)
Not	2	

IF TEETH FILLED (1)
(a) Have you ever had an injection in your gum to kill the pain of a filling?

Injection in gum	1
Not	2

(b) Have you ever had an injection in your arm to kill the pain of a filling?

Injection in arm	1
Not	2

120

(a) Have you ever had gas to have teeth taken out?

Had gas	1
Not	2

(b) Have you ever had an injection in your gum to have teeth taken out?

Injection in gum ...	1
Not	2

(c) Have you ever had an injection in your arm to have teeth taken out?

Injection in arm ...	1
Not	2

121 Have you ever had an X ray taken of your teeth?

Had X ray	1
Not	2

122 While you had your own teeth did you go to the dentist for regular check ups, occasional check ups or only when you had trouble with your teeth?

Regular check ups ..	1
Occasional check ups	2
Only when had trouble with teeth	3

Questions 123-127   DNA

14

112

131 (Can I just check) during the visit(s) you made to the dentist for that course of treatment did you have ......

INDIVIDUAL PROMPT

	YES	NO	DK
... Any Xrays taken	..1	2	3
Any teeth extracted	..1	2	3
Fitting of new dentures	..1	2	3
Repair of old dentures	..1	2	3
Any other treatment .... (SPECIFY)	..1	2	3

132 Was your treatment under the National Health Service, was it private or was it something else?

National Health Service .	1	ask(b)
Private	2	ask(a-b)
N.H.S. and private	3	
Community Dental Service.	4	
Armed Forces	5	
Other (SPECIFY)	6	

IF NHS AND PRIVATE (3)
(a) What treatment did you have privately?

IF ANY PRIVATE (2 or 3)
(b) What was the main reason for you having this treatment done privately?

133 How much did the treatment cost you?

Cost (SPECIFY)	1	ask(a)
Nothing	2	ask(b)
DK	3	go to Q.134

IF PAID FOR TREATMENT (1)
(a) Did the treatment cost more than you expected, about what you expected or less than you expected

More than expected	1	go to Q.134
About what expected ...	2	
Less than expected	3	
Other (SPECIFY)	4	

IF NOTHING (2)
(b) Why didn't it cost you anything?

PROMPT AS NEC.

No treatment	1	go to Q.134
Under 21, pregnant or nursing mother	2	ask(c)
Other (SPECIFY)	3	

(c) When you went to the dentist did you expect the treatment would be free?

Yes	1
No	2

16

134 Thinking about the dental practice you went to for your last treatment, was that the first time you had been to that dentist or group of dentists or had you been there before?

First time ...	1	ask (d)
Been before ..	2	ask (a-d)

IF BEEN BEFORE (2)
(a) For about how many years have you been going to that dentist or group of dentists?

Less than a year	1
One year less than two	2
Two years less than five ...	3
Five years or more	4
DK/Can't remember	5

(d) Last time you wanted to see the dentist about how long did you have to wait for an appointment?

135 How did you come to choose that particular dentist?

Can't remember ..	9

17

113

136 In the last five years have you had any difficulty in getting any treatment under the National Health Service?

Had difficulty 1
Not .... 2 ask (a-b)

IF HAD DIFFICULTY (1)
(a) What treatment couldn't you get?

ALL OF IT/
PART OF IT
IF PART WHAT PART?

(b) What did you do about it?

Questions 137 and 138 DNA

I'd like to talk generally now about the cost of dental treatment under the National Health Service.

139 When you go to the dentist to have treatment do you normally have some idea of how much it's going to cost you?

Has some idea 1
Does not .... 2 ask (a)

140 Do you know where you can find out about National Health Service dental charges?

Yes 1
No 2

IF YES
(a) Where can you find out?

Dentist 1
G.P.O. 2
Other (SPECIFY) ... 3

141 When you have to pay at the dentist does he usually tell you what the total cost is made up of?

Yes 1
No 2
Never paid 3

142 I'd like you to look at these different treatments and tell me how much you think each would cost, whether it would cost nothing or whether it would cost £2 or less, between £2 and £5, or £5 or more?

SHOW CARDS B AND C

	TREATMENT WOULD COST (C)				
COURSE OF TREATMENT (B)	Nothing (Free)	£2 or less	Between £2 & £5	£5 or more	DK
Exam, 2 teeth out	1	2	3	4	5
Exam, 1 large filling, 1 tooth out	1	2	3	4	5
Examination only	1	2	3	4	5
Exam, 2 Xrays, scale and polish, 1 small filling	1	2	3	4	5
Exam, 4 teeth out, new dentures fitted	1	2	3	4	5
Exam, 2 Xrays, 6 teeth out, gas	1	2	3	4	5
Repair of cracked denture	1	2	3	4	5
Exam, 2 Xrays, scale and polish ...	1	2	3	4	5

143 For the most kinds of treatment under the National Health Service the patient pays the full cost up to the first £5

(a) As a maximum charge do you think £5 is ...

	... too high	1
RUNNING	about right	2
PROMPT	or too low?	3

(b) A few kinds of dental treatment are rather expensive and so the patient has to pay more than £5 to be treated under the National Health Service.

Do you know what kinds of treatment cost the patient more than £5?

Yes 1   ask (c)
No 2

IF YES (1)
(c) What kinds of treatment cost the patient more than £5?

144 Some people get exemption from dental charges so that all the treatment they have is free.
Do you know what kinds of people get free treatment?

Yes 1   ask (a)
No 2

IF YES (1)
(a) What kinds of people get free treatment?

Pregnant or nursing mothers 1
Other (SPECIFY) 2

20

145 People have mentioned all sorts of things that make them put off going to the dentist. Can you look at this card and tell me for each of the statements I read out whether these things apply to you very much, a fair amount, not very much or not at all.

SHOW CARD D

APPLIES TO ME

I put off going to the dentist because	very much	a fair amount	not very much	not at all	DK
... I'm scared of the dentist	1	2	3	4	5
... It's difficult to get time off work	1	2	3	4	5
... It's too expensive to go too often	1	2	3	4	5
... I haven't got a regular dentist....	1	2	3	4	5
... I can't be bothered really........	1	2	3	4	5
... It's difficult to get an appointment......	1	2	3	4	5
... It's a long way to go.............	1	2	3	4	5

146 What do you find most unpleasant about going to the dentist?

147 Are there any other comments you would like to make about having false teeth?

21

CLASSIFICATION – TO ALL

150 (a) **Date of birth of informant**

Day	Month	Year

(b) **Sex of informant**

Male 1
Female .. 2

(c) **Age informant finished full time education**

14 years or less .. 4
15 years 5
16 years 6
17 years 7
18 years or more .. 8
Still in f/t education .. 9

(d) **Employment status of informant**

Full time 1
Part time 2
Not in employment .. 3

(e) **Marital status of informant**

Married 1
Single 2
W/S/D 3

(f) **What is the occupation of the informant?**
(GIVE OCCUPATION AND INDUSTRY)

(g) **IS THE INFORMANT HOH OR NOT?**

Informant HOH 1
Not 2   go to Q 151

151 **What is the occupation of the HOH?**
(GIVE OCCUPATION AND INDUSTRY)

116

22

Printed in England for Her Majesty's Stationery Office
by Commercial Colour Press, London E.7.
Dd.697911 K12 6/80